Ballistocardiography: Research and Computer Diagnosis

Proceedings of the 16th Annual Meeting of the Ballistocardiograph Research Society
Atlantic City, N.J., April 1972

Ballistocardiography: Research and Computer Diagnosis

Editor: Ernst K. Franke
Department of Physics, University of Cincinnati, Cincinnati, Ohio

With 71 figures and 14 tables

1973

S. Karger · Basel · München · Paris · London · New York · Sydney

Bibliotheca Cardiologica, No. 32

Ballistocardiography and Clinical Studies
Proceedings of the 14th Annual Meeting of the Ballistocardiograph Research Society,
Atlantic City, N.J., May 1970
Edited by W.K. Harrison
VIII + 84 p., 33 fig., 8 tab., 1971 (Bibliotheca Cardiologica, No. 27)
ISBN 3-8055-1188-4

Circulatory Assists and Ballistocardiographic Studies
Proceedings of the 15th Annual Meeting of the Ballistocardiograph Research Society,
Atlantic City, N.J., 1971
Edited by D.H. Jackson
VI + 114 p., 55 fig., 4 tab., 1972 (Bibliotheca Cardiologica, No. 29)
ISBN 3-8055-1323-2

Proceedings of the 8th European Congress on Ballistocardiography and Cardiovascular Dynamics, Ljubljana, April 1971
Editor: G. Južnič, Ljubljana
Part I: Lectures
Hemodynamic Stress and Relief of the Heart
XII + 159 p., 65 fig., 13 tab., 1973 (Bibliotheca Cardiologica, No. 30)
ISBN 3-8055-1374-7
Part II: Free Communications
Biomedical Science and Cardiovascular Dynamics
(Bibliotheca Cardiologica No. 31)
ISBN 3-8055-1375-5

S. Karger · Basel · München · Paris · London · New York · Sydney
Arnold-Böcklin-Strasse 25, CH-4011 Basel (Switzerland)

Printed in Switzerland by Basler Druck- und Verlagsanstalt, Basel
Blocks: Steiner & Co., Basel
ISBN 3-8055-1376-3

Table of Contents

Preface

The papers published in this volume were presented at the 16th Annual meeting of the U. S. Ballistocardiograph Research Society on April 29, 1972, in Atlantic City, New Jersey. Their content is almost evenly divided among clinical applications, biophysical research, and computer aided interpretation. Among the recent developments which are reflected in their titles is the growing recognition and accumulation of evidence that the ballistocardiogram, and especially its initial part, is a useful measure of myocardial function and a welcome addition to other methods of its quantification. If only for this reason the ballistocardiogram will be of growing importance to multiphasic health screening. It combines the advantages of non-invasiveness, easy application, and proven prognostic sensitivity. The profusion of data which must be expected to accumulate in health screening activities will make computer aided interpretation a necessity. Substantial progress toward this goal is demonstrated by contributors to this volume. The high quality of the papers is undeniable evidence of the important role which ballistocardiography is destined to play in early recognition of heart disease, and proof that it deserves continuing research support. It should, finally, not be left unmentioned that this volume marks another memorable event: the whale has joined man, dog and turtle as a subject for ballistocardiographic research. As is becoming for a young, female representative of the species, her ballistocardiogram is quite normal by human standards.

E. K. Franke, Editor

Proc. 16th ann. Meet. Ballistocard. Res. Soc., Atlantic City 1972;
Bibl. Cardiol. *32:* 1–10 (Karger, Basel 1973)

Automatic Computer Processing of Ultralow Frequency Ballistocardiograms[1]

W. H. Bancroft, jr., Marjorie Tucker, D. H. Jackson and E. E. Eddleman, jr.

Veterans Administration Hospital and Department of Medicine,
University of Alabama School of Medicine, Birmingham, Ala.

Recent studies have shown the ultralow frequency ballistocardiogram (Bcg) to be a very sensitive early indicator of heart disease [1–6]. In order to facilitate comprehensive investigation of this procedure of early detection, a rapid method of waveform recognition has been developed. The procedure requires the Frank lead vectorcardiogram followed by simultaneous recordings of the Y lead, the carotid pulse pressure, and the ultralow frequency Bcg. It is the purpose of this paper to describe a system that has been designed to automatically prepare these data by computer for further analysis.

Method

The ballistocardiographic system consists of an ultralow frequency air-bearing bed made and designed at Johns Hopkins University. The accelerometer is a Northam Model A-14 with a range of ± 0.5 g and measures the acceleration in the head-foot direction only. The transducer is connected to an Electronics for Medicine Model SGA-6 pressure amplifier and a DR-8 recorder. Each ballistocardiographic recording is preceded by a calibration consisting of a square wave which is derived from the steps of the pressure amplifier. This square wave is periodically calibrated in cm/sec^2 units using an eccentric weight mounted on a synchronous motor fastened to the bed. The data are stored on a 1-inch analog magnetic tape employing an Ampex 14-channel FR-1300 recorder.

The system consists of a Digital Equipment Corporation PDP-8 which is connected through the data break to a Xerox Data Systems Sigma-7 computer operating in a time-sharing mode. The operator may choose analog signals coming directly from the patient, or from an analog tape. The signals are displayed on a 5-inch, 4-channel oscilloscope, and after viewing the patient and curve identifications are typed in at the request of the com-

[1] Aided by VA Research Funds and USPH grant No. HE-11310 and 5 PO7 RR00145-09.

puter program. When a useable portion is identified, analog to digital conversion is started by depressing a key on the teletype. The resultant digital curves are displayed back on a Tektronix 611 memory oscilloscope. Data are converted at a rate of 250 samples per second per channel for a total of 8000 samples per channel, or 3.2 sec.

The program requires the operator to accept or reject the data. If acceptable, they are transmitted to the Sigma-7 computer where they are transferred to a disc for further manipulation. The procedure is as follows:

The operator digitizes a 2-mV square wave to calibrate the X, Y, Z leads. Then these data are transmitted to the XDS computer. The X, Y, Z leads are digitized, accepted and transferred to the Sigma-7 computer where the beginning of the QRS complex (Q) is determined. Figure 1 describes the method for locating Q and the time from Q to the peak of the R wave (R). Next, the ballistocardiographic calibration is digitized. The step size is determined by the program, stored, and then the Bcg is digitized. Both held inspiration and held expiration are routinely processed.

Figure 2 shows the carotid, Y-lead and Bcg reproduced from the DR-8 recording. Methods of determining the Q, carotid upstroke (CU) and carotid incisural notch (CIN) are indicated. This procedure rarely fails on Q or CU. It is accurate approximately 85% of the time on CIN. The procedure fails more often on curves from patients with hypertrophic subaortic stenosis. The Sigma-7 transfers these locations back to the PDP-8 where they are displayed on the memory oscilloscope, and the operator has the option to accept or reject. If rejection is chosen, the locations can be changed by typing a direction and

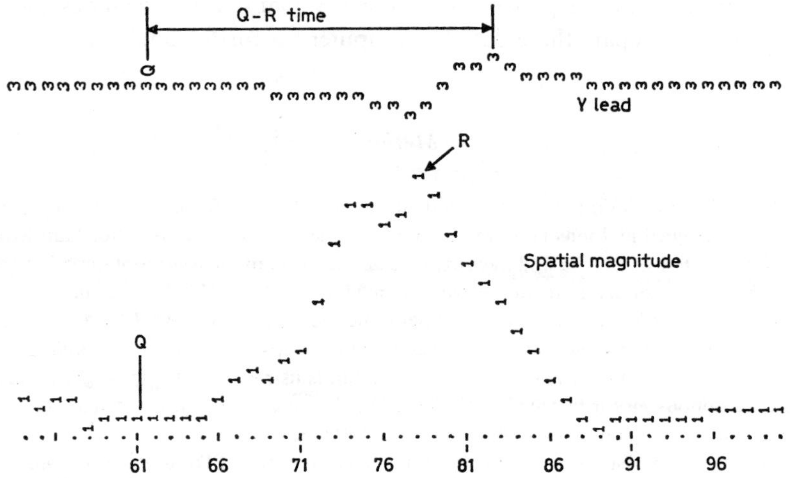

Fig. 1. Location of Q and Q-R time: (1) Locate R (peak) on spatial magnitude (filtered with 3 point sliding filter and calibrated). (2) Move to left to find 5 slopes (2 points) in a row whose amplitudes are ±1 mV/msec. (3) Move to right and find first slope greater than 2 mV/msec. (4) This point is defined as 'Q'. (5) Determine if Y lead is positive going or negative going. (6) Find R-peak on Y lead and compute Q-R time. (7) Repeat for 3 complexes and find average Q-R time.

magnitude for each of the points (for example, typing CU2-030 moves the location of the second upstroke to the left 30 points). When all corrections are made, the operator types 'K'.

The next procedure is to deslope the Bcg. Figure 3 illustrates why this is sometimes necessary and how it is done. This is a recording made while the ballistocardiographic

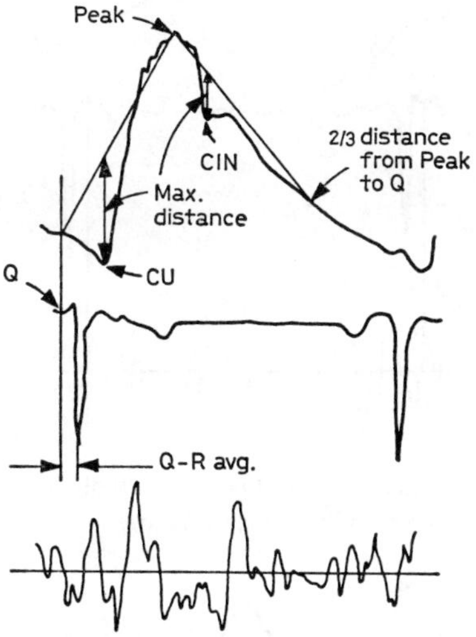

Fig. 2. Location of Q, CU and CIN: (1) Locate R on Y lead. (2) Subtract Q-R average from location of R; this is Q. (3) Assume line from Q time on carotid pulse to peak. (4) Location of maximum distance from line to curve is CU. (5) Assume line from peak to $^2/_3$ distance from peak to next Q on carotid. (6) Location of maximum distance from line to curve is CIN.

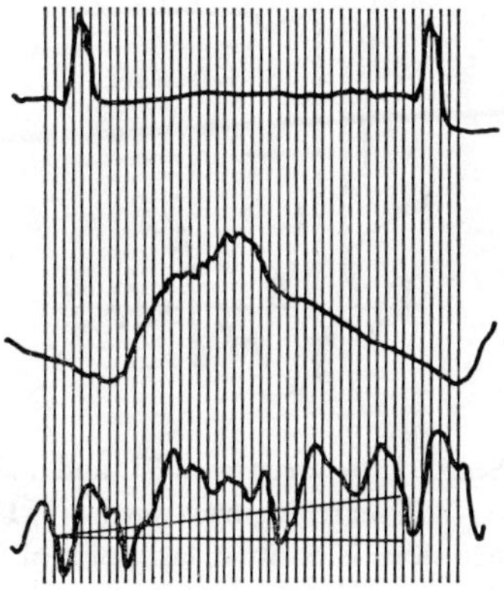

Fig. 3. Deslope: (1) Each complex is 'desloped' individually from Q to Q. (2) A straigth line error is assumed. (3) A sine for tangent approximation is made.

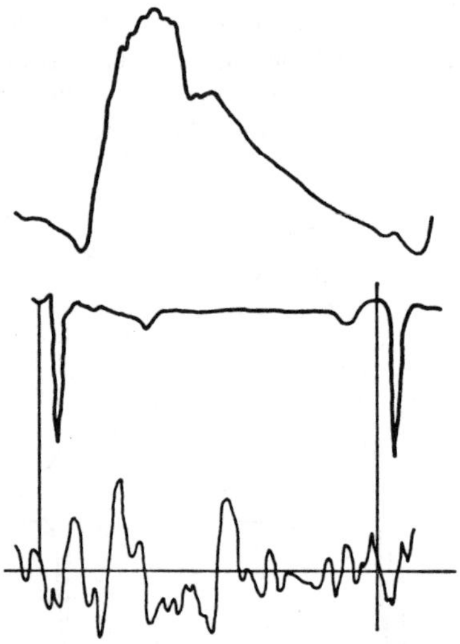

Fig. 4. Determining baseline. The baseline is established by requiring the area above the zero acceleration line to be equal to the area below.

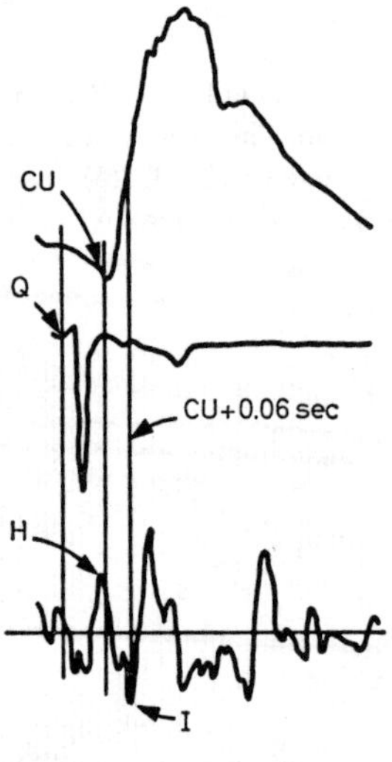

Fig. 5. Find H and I. (1) Search backwards from CU and find first positive value. (2) Find first positive slope (2 points) – still searching backwards. (3) Find average slope (2 points) of next 8 points. (4) If average slope is positive, last point of first positive slope is defined as H. (5) If average is negative, start search back one point and repeat procedure. (6) If these criteria cannot be met in interval between Q and CU, define H as highest point in the interval. (7) 'I' is defined as the lowest point in the interval between H and CU +0.06 sec.

bed was swinging, showing a sloping curve. It probably would be rejected as an unacceptable complex; however, it is made useable by the desloping procedure.

Figure 4 illustrates the use of the conservation of energy theorem to determine the baseline. For the isolated system during one heartbeat the sum of the forces in the headward direction must equal the sum of the forces in the footward direction. This requires the areas above and below the baseline to be equal for each complex. The program assumes a baseline half way between the maximum and minimum points on the ballistocardiographic curve. It computes the area above and the area below the baseline, calculates half the difference, and divides this by the number of points. This establishes the distance which the baseline is moved so that the areas become equal.

Figure 5 points out how H and I are located. Throughout this discussion the letters used indicate the peak of the wave. For example, 'H' is the peak of the H wave. Figure 6 illustrates the location of first J. Figure 7 describes location of K. Figure 8 describes the location of other J's. A digital tape is made of these data and further computation is done in the 'batch' mode. Figure 9 shows a scattergram plot of one complex for a given patient with locations as found by the program. Further computations are performed in the 'batch' mode and list the following averaged measurements for each patient:

Amplitudes: H, I, HI, J1, IJ1, J2, J3, K.

Durations: Q-H, Q-I, Q-J1, Q-K, H-I, I-J1, I-J2, Q-CU, CU-CIN, Heart Rate.

Slopes: H-I, H′-I, I-J, I-J′. The point H′ is defined as that point on the ballistocardiographic curve which first crosses the baseline by searching backwards from I toward H. Similarly, J′ is located by searching forward from I-J to find the first point on the ballisto-

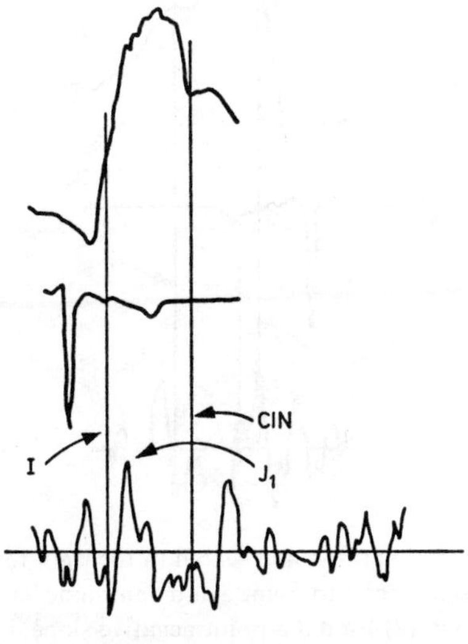

Fig. 6. Find first J. (1) Begin at I or CU, whichever is latest, and search to CIN for a 2-point negative slope. (2) Find average of next four slopes (2 point). (3) If this average is negative and the peak is a positive amplitude, the peak is first J. (4) If slope is not negative, move starting point one point to the right and repeat the procedure.

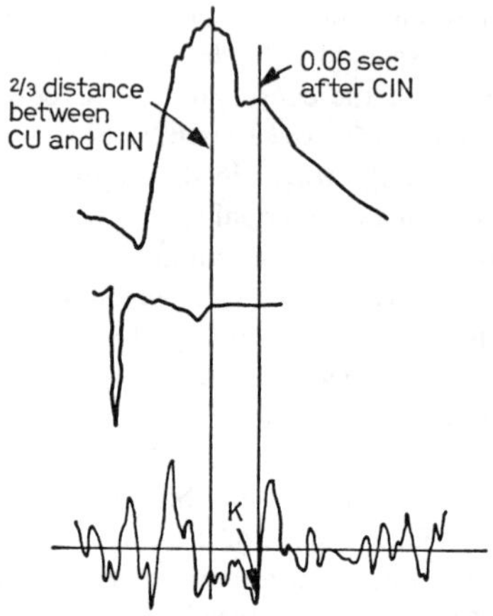

Fig. 7. Find K. Search from point $^2/_3$ distance between CU and CIN to 0.06 sec after CIN for lowest point. This is defined as 'K'.

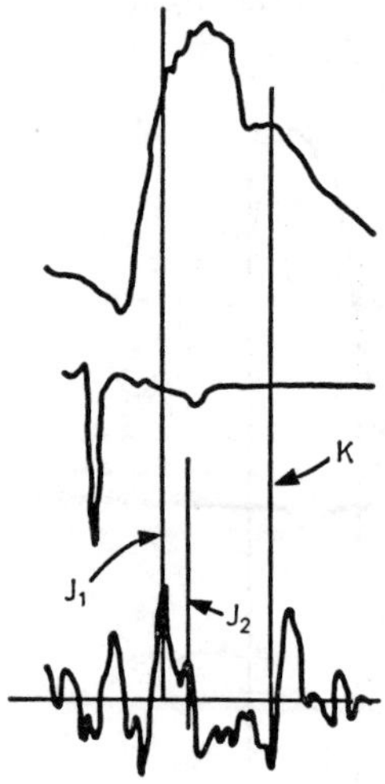

Fig. 8. Find next J. (1) Begin at first and search to the right for a positive 5-point slope. (Assume a straight line from point 1 to point 5 and determine its slope.) The search ends at K or CIN, whichever is first. (2) Find a 5-point negative slope. (3) Test to see if first point of the negative slope is a positive number. (4) If this number is positive, the point is defined as next J. Routine allows for 5-J waves by repeating the search from location of J_1. (5) If this number is negative, the search is repeated beginning at the location of the point of the negative slope.

cardiographic curve that crosses the baseline. These points are believed to be more definitive for determining slopes.

A test was made to determine the accuracy of the ballistocardiographic amplitudes as found by the computer. Amplitudes were measured by hand on ballistocardiographic plots of a series of patients (7 with aortic stenosis and 17 normal). By comparison, the results of the IJ amplitude measurements are shown in figure 10. The correlation coefficient was 0.985.

Discussion

There are a number of arbitrary decisions that must be made before any waveform recognition program can be implemented. For example, the criteria

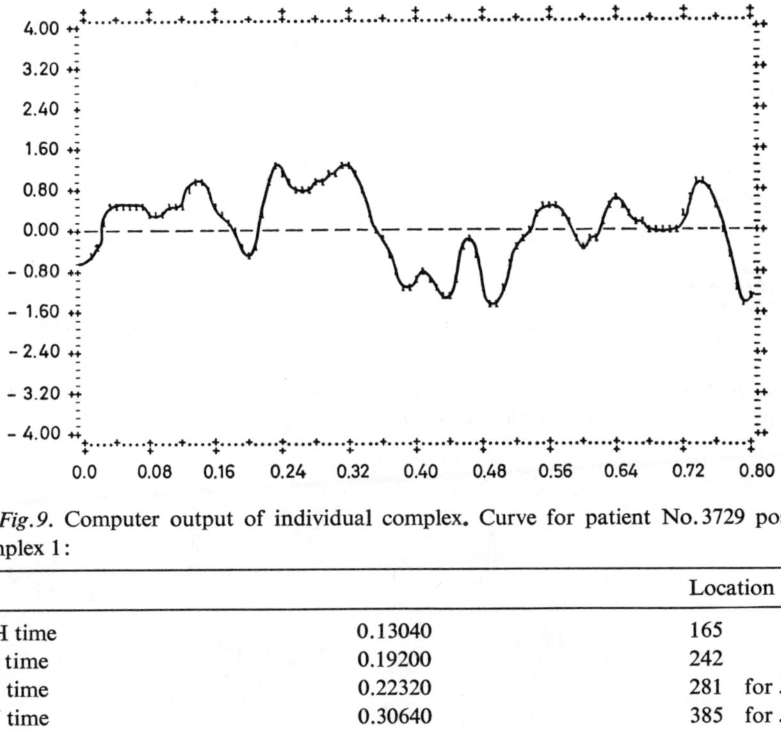

Fig.9. Computer output of individual complex. Curve for patient No. 3729 pos. 98 complex 1:

		Location	
Q-H time	0.13040	165	
Q-I time	0.19200	242	
Q-J time	0.22320	281	for J1
Q-J time	0.30640	385	for J2
Q-K time	0.42640	535	
Q-CU time	0.13040	165	for CU
CU-CIN time	0.30160	542	for CIN
Q-Q heartrate	66.19592		

for locating H as described requires H to be located prior to the carotid upstroke. On several occasions, a cardiologist has selected a point which appears after the carotid upstroke, as shown in figure 11. Since the computer is consistent and does not search past the carotid upstroke, it finds a small projection as H at an earlier location. Which is the more accurate selection?

Occasionally, an H will swap positions in time from complex to complex for a given patient. For example, an earlier small projection will appear

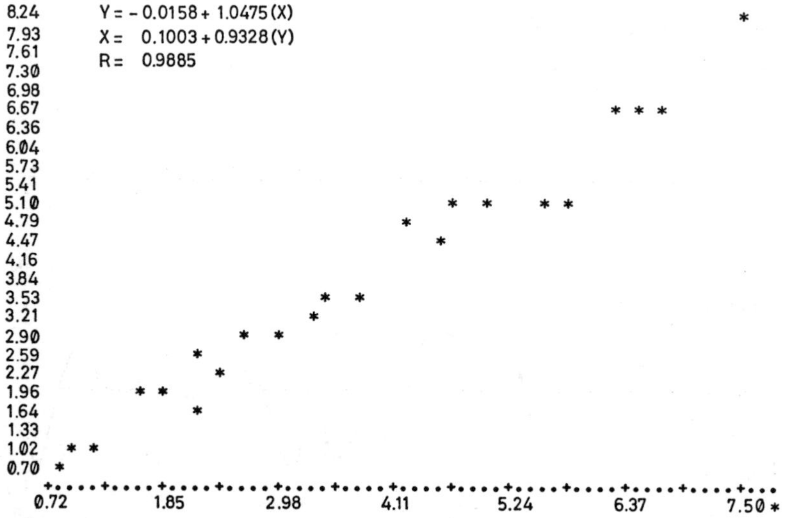

Fig. 10. Correlation of hand measurements (Y) and computer measurements (X). Units are cm/sec². Equations are simple regression.

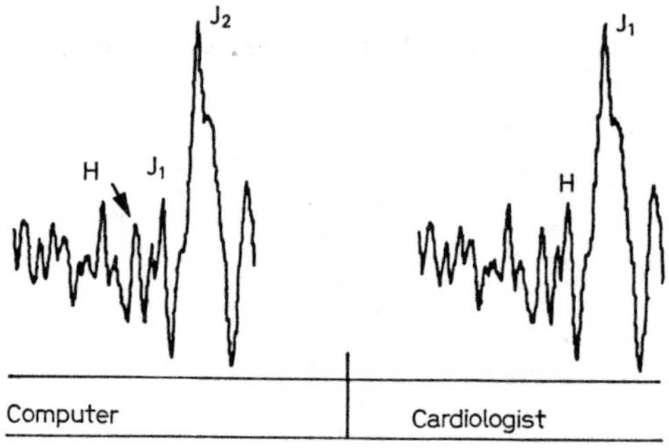

Fig. 11. H found by cardiologist comes after CU. Computer location is on left.

prominently in the next complex and cause the H to be identified in a different place. This same type problem also can occur with I and J. The question which needs to be resolved is whether these are artefacts in the ballistocardiographic system or whether they are actual physiological changes. At this time there are no answers, but by recording several patients with a large number of complexes, observing the variations, and attempting to determine whether they are random in nature or periodic may be useful in determining a solution to the question. At this time it may be a necessity to either make measurements on a large number of individual complexes and compute the mean or average many complexes to form one waveform before making the measurements. These problems point out the need for better criteria as to waveform definitions.

The process of making the complete procedure automatic is in progress. The locations of the points on the Bcg will be determined by the XDS computer and displayed back on the storage scope. The operator will verify or move the locations as in the procedure for finding the upstroke and notch on the carotid pulse. The present on-line system for locating the Q, CU and CIN records both the locations found by the computer and the new locations determined by the operator. A similar procedure will be available in the new program and will give a method for evaluating the computer results as compared to that of a trained operator.

Summary

A method for rapid processing of ballistocardiograms has been developed for use of recorded signals on analog magnetic tape or with data coming directly from a patient. For a group of 24 patients, each with two to three complexes available, the I-J amplitudes were measured by hand and by computer. The correlation coefficient between the two was 0.985. Variations in waveforms from beat to beat suggest further studies are needed to determine whether or not they are due to physiologic variations or artefacts in the system. In the meantime, many complexes should be used to eliminate random artefacts.

References

1 Starr, I.: On the later development of heart disease in apparently healthy persons with abnormal ballistocardiograms. Eight- to ten-year after-histories of 90 persons over 40 years of age. Amer. J. med. Sci. *214:* 233–242 (1947).

2 Starr, I.: Prognostic value of ballistocardiograms. Studies on evaluation of the doctor's experience. J. amer. med. Ass. *187:* 511–517 (1964).

3 STARR, I.; ASKOVITZ, S.I., and MANDELBAUM, E.M.: Items of prognostic value in the clinical study; the relationship of symptoms, heart size, blood-pressure, electrocardiogram, and ballistocardiogram to after-histories and to each other. J. amer. med. Ass. *192:* 83–87 (1965).

4 STARR, I.: Prognostic value of ballistocardiograms; as judged by after-histories of 211 healthy persons and 221 patients followed from 5 to 25 years. Proc. 1st World Congr. in Ballistocardiographic Cardiovascular Dynamics, Amsterdam 1965, pp. 7–20 (Karger, Basel 1966).

5 BAKER, B.M.; SCARBOROUGH, W.R.; DAVIS, F.W., jr.; MASON, R.E., and SINGWALL, M.L. (Statistical Evaluation: WALKER, S.H.; MURPHY, E.A.; HARRISON, W.K., jr., and SHERWIN, R.W.): Ballistocardiography and ischemic heart disease; predictive considerations and statistical evaluation. Proc. roy. Soc. Med. *60:* 1290–1296 (1967).

6 TAYLOR, H.L.; KEYS, A., and BLACKBURN, H.: The prognostic importance for coronary heart disease and death of the low-frequency critical damped ballistocardiogram: eighteen years of follow-up. Amer. J. Cardiol. (submitted, April 1972).

Author's address: Mr. WILLIAM H. BANCROFT, jr., Veterans Administration Hospital, 700 South 19th Street, *Birmingham AL 35233* (USA)

Proc. 16th ann. Meet. Ballistocard. Res. Soc., Atlantic City 1972;
Bibl. Cardiol. *32:* 11–14 (Karger, Basel 1973)

Computer Preprocessing of Ballistocardiograms

I. Tomek

Department of Medicine, The University of Alberta, Edmonton, Alberta

Introduction

At least two approaches to the computerized processing of Bcg's have been described so far [1, 2]. Both of them have two features which do not seem to make full use of the possibilities of computer processing and could thus be improved upon: (1) human participation in the preprocessing (namely the choice of cycles to be used in the main program of Bcg records) is necessary; (2) averaging of all chosen cycles is one of the basic characteristics of processing algorithms. It is not necessary to discuss the desirability of the elimination of human participation. As for averaging, it is well known that especially Bcg's of abnormal subjects very often contain patterns not resembling one another or forming groups of similar patterns (usually related to breathing). When this is the case, however, it is difficult to justify overall averaging; it can lead to a significant loss of information since the 'average' patterns may not resemble any of the patterns actually present in the processed record. The most straight forward way of avoiding this danger is to cluster the various patterns according to their shapes before averaging and average only over individual clusters. Representation of clusters by these averages and representation of the whole record by typical patterns thus found, and also possibly some other information of statistical nature could thus both reduce the amount of data to be processed later and preserve much of the original information. This information about a given Bcg could then be used to classify the record by comparison with a library of information about normal and abnormal Bcg's. This library, however, does not exist yet and there is not enough knowledge to set up a set of rules to classify records directly from the information described above. The first application of a program capable of handling Bcg records in this way is thus to serve as an objective tool in the process of the building of this collection.

Description of the Program

In the first part of the program, individual cycles are identified. For this purpose, the point of maximum slope in the Q-R interval of the ECG is used. Since the systolic part is believed to contain most information (also to decide upon the similarity of patterns as short intervals as possible are desirable) each cycle is represented by an interval beginning at this point and .4 sec long. A set of patterns is thus obtained from the whole record. This set of patterns is then processed by a routine designed for this purpose and described by TOMEK [3]. Its goal is the identification of groups of similar records contained in the processed record. It resolves both the problems mentioned in the introduction since it automatically discards patterns affected by artefacts and patterns atypical for the given record. It works essentially as follows:

(1) Each pattern is represented by a set of N numbers. Fourier coefficients have been used for this purpose successfully (fig. 1) but other representations are being investigated.

(2) Each pattern is associated with a group of similar patterns contained in the examined record. This step is based upon distance of points in an N-

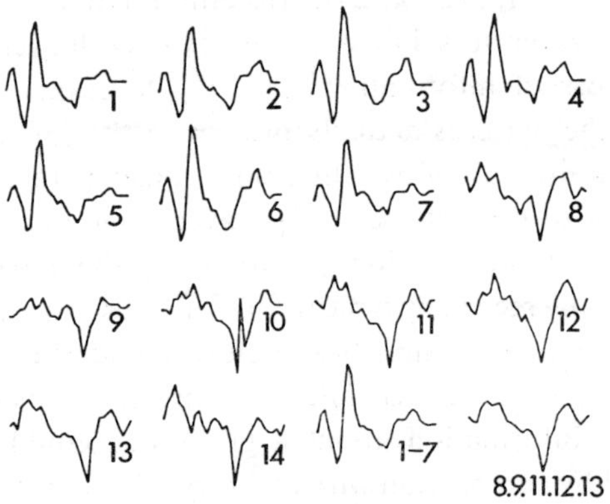

Fig. 1. An example of the extraction of typical patterns. Patterns 1–7 are found to be similar. Also 8, 9, 11, 12, 13 are similar. These two groups are represented by the last two patterns at lower right. Patterns 10, 14 are not members of any of these two groups.

dimensional space; patterns (points) closer than L (limit of similarity found by comparison in the subjective judgement) are considered as similar.

(3) All clusters thus obtained (containing enough points) are assigned weights depending upon their densities (intra-cluster distances) and the number of points in the cluster.

(4) The cluster with the maximum weight is accepted as a representative group and eliminated from further considerations. Also eliminated are clusters too close to this accepted group. This step is repeated until no further clusters remain for processing.

In the next stage, averages of obtained groups are calculated and accepted as patterns representative of the given record.

Incorporation of other features (e.g. of statistical character) is considered for the latter stages of development of this program.

Conclusion

The program described above is an expression of the author's belief that classification of Bcg's by their shapes is possible and gives hope of better discrimination of abnormalities than the usual approach requiring identification of various peaks, measurement of amplitudes and slopes. It is based on the fact that the Bcg is the result of a complex interaction of the contraction of the heart and the distributed system of blood vessels. It is an output of a system with distributed parameters. Its individual peaks in general do not represent uniquely identifiable events in the heart cycle. (Also these peaks are often difficult or impossible to identify.) This makes the Bcg different from the ECG which is basically an output of a system with 'lumped' elements. For this reason methods used for ECG evaluation (location of peaks and measurements) may not be optimal for the Bcg. It may be that a combination of the standard approach and evaluation by comparison of shapes of Bcg's would be the best method. For this purpose many Bcg's must be recorded and processed and various approaches tried, modified and perhaps combined. Standardization of recording and cooperation of Bcg users would be most helpful in this project.

Summary

This paper describes an approach to computerized preprocessing of ballistocardiograms (Bcg). It differs from methods described elsewhere in two main points: (1) it is completely automatic – processing of a digitized record does not require any human intervention or supervision; (2) individual Bcg waveforms in each record are grouped into sets of similar patterns (patterns which cannot be classified as belonging to any large group of similar records are eliminated from further processing). The last feature makes it possible to obtain one or several patterns 'typical' for a given record – typical records are defined as averages of patterns in individual groups. These typical patterns can either be stored to become members of a library of typical Bcg's (this is the present use – preprocessing) or used for computerized classification of a given record by comparison with a library of normal and abnormal Bcg's (processing – this is the ultimate reason for the creation of the library).

References

1 HARRISON, W.K.; BURTON, M.E., and GLASPELL, F.: Computer analysis of ballistocardiograms. Comput. biomed. Res. *5:* 279–290 (1972).
2 BANCROFT, W.H. *et al.:* Bibl. cardiol., vol. 32, pp. 1–10 (Karger, Basel 1973).
3 TOMEK, I.: Comput. biomed. Res. (to be published).

Author's address: I. TOMEK, Department of Medicine, The University of Alberta, *Edmonton,* Alberta

Proc. 16th ann. Meet. Ballistocard. Res. Soc., Atlantic City 1972;
Bibl. Cardiol. *32:* 15–21 (Karger, Basel 1973)

A Large-Scale Model of the Human Cardiovascular System and its Application to Ballistocardiography

D. M. Auslander, T. E. Lobdell and D. Chong

Mechanical Engineering Department, University of California, Berkeley, Calif.,
and General Motors Technical Center, Warren, Mich.,
and General Electric Company, San Jose, Calif.

Introduction

Although pressure pulse propagation in mammalian cardiovascular systems immediately suggests the use of distributed-parameter models, previous work [1, 2] has been concentrated in the construction of large and small-scale lumped-parameter models in which segments of the system are modeled with RLC networks. Both analog and digital computers have been used to solve the system equations derived for these models.

We feel that digital computer realizations or large-scale models can achieve the most flexibility and usability. Therefore, we have approached this problem by constructing a digital model based on distributed-parameter dynamic elements, thereby increasing the computation efficiency somewhat and introducing a better model at the segment-by-segment level.

Through the use of an already existing general purpose bond-graph simulation program we were able to proceed to the simulation and testing of the model without the necessity of writing or solving any equations. In this program, which we call DBOND, all of the system dynamics are described by ideal bilateral transmission lines [3] called delay-bonds. System topology is represented by a bond graph in which delay-bonds are interconnected by static junctions.

Our goal in building the cardiovascular system model was to show that it is possible to build a model that is physiologically pure enough and computationally flexible enough to be a general research tool and, ultimately, perhaps even a clinical tool. We were aided in the attainment of physiological purity by the fact that a transmission line is described by a length, a wave speed and a characteristic impedance, parameters that correspond closely to normal anatomical and physiological parameters, especially in the arterial system. In computing program inputs we used only primary data, supported by previous research, unless such data were simply not available.

The flexibility of our model was tested in an attempt to help determine the clinical significance of ballistocardiogram records. The use of large-scale simulation was proposed because it is impossible at present to get experimental correlation on a human subject between the large number of internal states of the cardiovascular system and a Bcg.

Vascular and Heart Models

A delay-bond graph of the cardiovascular model is shown in figure 1. The lines in the graph stand for ideal, bilateral transmission lines [3], each characterized by a wave transit time and a characteristic impedance. The circled nodes represent static system characteristics such as resistance and sources. In most cases, each delay line accounts for the dynamics of one blood vessel. Sometimes two or more delay-lines are used to model area or property

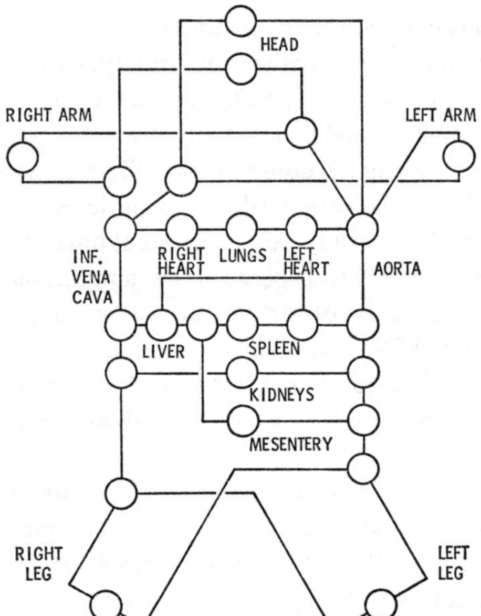

Fig. 1. Delay-bond graph of the cardiovascular model.

changes along the vessel. The resistance becomes incorporated into the junctions. The wave travel time, T, characteristic impedance, Z, and resistance, R, of a uniform segment of blood vessel were taken as [4]

$$T = \sqrt{IC} = \lambda(a+1) \left[\frac{3\rho}{E\,(2a+1)}\right]^{1/2}, \tag{1}$$

$$Z = \sqrt{I/C} = \frac{1}{S\,(a+1)} \left[{}^{1}/_{3}\,\rho\,E\,(2a+1)\right]^{1/2}, \tag{2}$$

$$R = \frac{8\,\pi\,\mu\,\lambda}{S^2},$$

where I = total distributed inertance; C = total distributed compliance; μ = blood viscosity (taken equal to 3×10^{-2} poise); ϱ = blood density (1.05 g cm^{-3}); S = internal cross-sectional area; a = ratio of internal vessel radius to vessel wall thickness; λ = segment length; E = Young's modulus.

Sixty-three systemic arterial vessels of internal diameter greater than approximately 0.10 cm were modeled by 110 segments, using data drawn mostly from WESTERHOF *et al.* [5]. Fifty-three systemic veins were represented in the model by 65 segments. Due to lack of data, the characteristics of these vessels were estimated from those of systemic arteries using assumptions regarding modulus of elasticity and relative dimensions. Systemic vessels of internal diameter of less than 0.1 cm were grouped together with the appropriate capillary bed, and were modeled as resistance-free compliant mixing tanks. The peripheral resistances were calculated to give prescribed bed pressures and flows.

The ventricles of the left and right hearts were modeled by delay lines whose compliances varied with time. This simulation method is based on one presented by BENEKEN [6]. Each ventricle was considered to be a compliant cylinder closed at one end. The compliance of the cylinder decreases along with its volume during the ejection phase of heart operation according to equations 1 and 2 which relate compliance and cross-sectional area. Passive lines were used to model the atria. The valves were modeled by resistive junctions whose resistances changed in response to the sign of the pressure differential across them. Ventricular parameters were set at values which produced specified pressure-flow relationships in the vessels immediately connected to the heart. The time course of compliance variation during ejection was modified somewhat during the ballistocardiography studies.

Model Performance

Simulated pressure and flow histories in the heart and aorta are shown in figure 2 [for more detailed results, see 7]. These may be compared to measurements made by SNELL *et al.* [8] shown in figure 3. The wave velocities in various simulated arterial segments were found to be within 15% of that measured in the actual segments. As demonstrations of the generality and possible clinical/research use that might be made of the model, it was used to study fainting, embolism, and hypertension. Results of these studies are contained in reference 4.

Application to Ballistocardiography

In a separate project[1], we then turned to the simulation of the human ballistocardiogram (Bcg). The simulated Bcg is computed by applying con-

[1] This work was supported by an NIH Biomedical Sciences Support Grant, USPHS FR-7006-05-Biomedical Support.

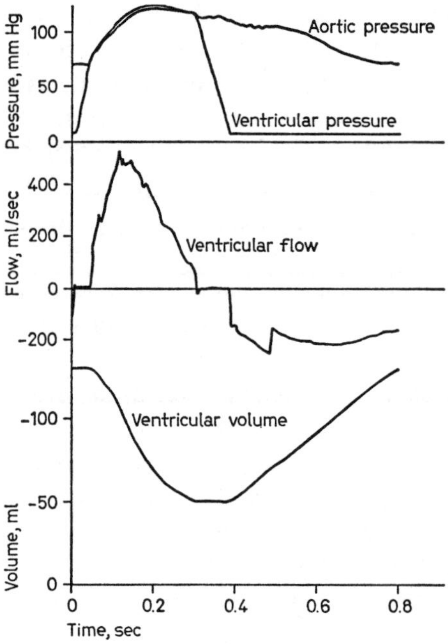

Fig. 2. Simulated pressure and flow histories in heart and aorta.

servation of momentum to the cardiovascular model; that is, we assume that the momentum attained by the blood in a given direction is most significant in the Bcg and causes an equal but opposite momentum to be imparted to the body. The velocity Bcg can be computed directly from this momentum; the displacement Bcg is obtained by integration and the acceleration Bcg by differentiation of the velocity record. Our method has the promise of giving better results than the center-of-mass technique [9] in which the displacement Bcg is produced directly and must be numerically differentiated twice, a very noisy and inaccurate procedure, to get the acceleration Bcg. In order to utilize the original cardiovascular model as a basis for this ballistocardiograph study, the only additional information required by the program was geo-

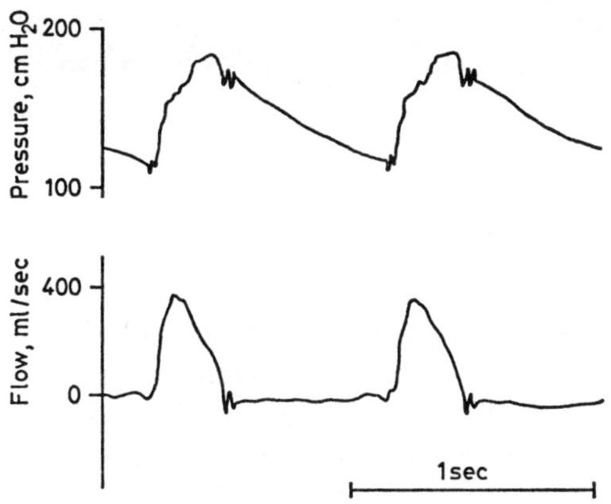

Fig. 3. Measured pressure and flow histories in the aorta [after SNELL *et al.*, 8].

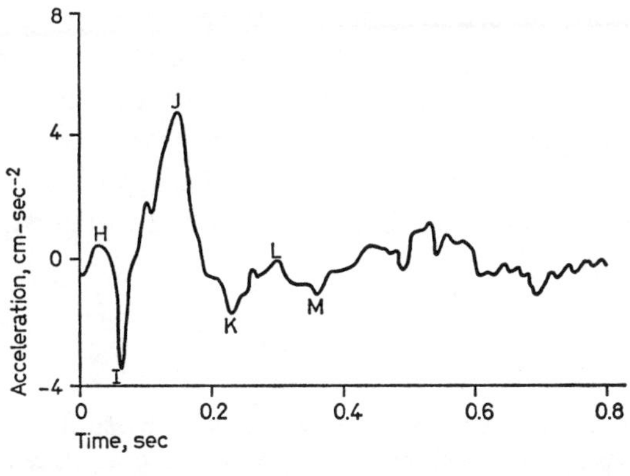

Fig. 4. Simulated acceleration or force ballistocardiograph.

metrical – the lengths and direction numbers of the vascular segments in the model. This new information was simply read into the program, and the ballistocardiograms then computed by a new subroutine. In addition, exponential smoothing was incorporated for the computation of the acceleration Bcg.

Before applying the simulation to ballistocardiography, the heart model was improved in order to bring the time derivative of the left ventricular pressure in to line with that shown in the literature [10].

The acceleration Bcg is given in figure 4. The result of the simulation shows that the characteristic HIJ wave is clearly present, though the K, L, M, and N waves are somewhat less distinct. Changes in the heart model to improve the ventricular pressure derivative (referred to above) had a marked effect on the Bcg, indicating the sensitivity of the Bcg to this characteristic. In the original case, the ratio of I wave to J wave amplitude was much smaller than normally expected (about ½). After modification, this ratio became nearly one, as can be seen in figure 4.

Conclusions

The results of this feasibility study demonstrate clearly that it is possible to use the DBOND cardiovascular simulation to obtain realistic simulated ballistocardiograms. The initial goal of building a cardiovascular model that could be used as a general-purpose research tool has at least been shown to be reasonable – at the time the model was constructed there was no thought of using it for Bcg's. The ease with which the model could be modified to compute Bcg's demonstrates its versatility and physiological homomorphism.

Further work on the basic model should be concentrated in two areas: improving the heart model and improving the representation of venous blood flow. Neither of these are pure modeling problems, however. Considerable basic physiological and engineering research is required to obtain a better understanding of what is going on. The ballistocardiography study was, of course, a feasibility study. Its success points the way towards further efforts at establishing the physiological significance of individual Bcg records.

Summary

Bond graphs have been used to construct a distributed-parameter model of the human cardiovascular system. The model includes the heart and arterial, capillary, and venous segments of both the pulmonary and systemic circulations. Anatomical and physiological data were utilized in implementing the model on a large digital computer. Comparisons of stimulated output and measured responses are shown.

Because a general-purpose bond graph simulation language for distributed-parameter systems was used, this cardiovascular simulation retains considerable flexibility and can be modified to suit the application. One such application that has been investigated in detail is the simulation of the body motions caused by blood flow in a subject mechanically isolated from the earth. This measurement, the ballistocardiogram (Bcg) holds the possibility of a non-invasive means of determining heart output.

Acknowledgements

Part of this work was supported by the NIH, through a research grant as noted in the paper and in the form of a Bioengineering Traineeship grant to Dr. T. LOBDELL.

We would like to gratefully acknowledge the assistance of Prof. D. M. CUNNINGHAM and Dr. A. G. DINABURG, M.D., for their help with the ballistocardiography studies.

References

1 NOORDERGRAAF, A.: Development of an analog computer for the human systemic circulatory system; in NOORDERGRAAF, JAGER and WESTERHOF Circulatory analog computers (North Holland Publishing Co., Amsterdam 1962).

2 ATTINGER, E. O. and ANNE, A.: Simulation of the cardiovascular system. Ann. N.Y. Acad. Sci. *128:* 810 (1966).

3 AUSLANDER, D. M.: Distributed system simulation with bilateral delay-line models. ASME Trans. J. Basic. Engineer. *90:* 195–200 (1968).

4 LOBDELL, T. E.: A digital computer model of the cardiovascular system; Engineer. Diss., Mechanical Engineering Department, University of California, Berkeley (1970).

5 WESTERHOF, N.; BOSMAN, F.; DEVRIES, C. J., and NOORDERGRAAF, A.: Analog studies of the human systemic arterial tree. J. Biomech. *2:* 121 (1969).

6 BENEKEN, J.E.W.: A mathematical approach to cardiovascular function; Ph.D. Thesis, Institute of Medical Physics, Utrecht (1965).

7 AUSLANDER, D. M.; LOBDELL, T. E., and CHONG, D.: A large-scale model of the human cardiovascular system and its application to ballistocardiography. ASME Trans. J. Dynamic Systems, Measurement, and Control, September 1972.

8 SNELL, R. E. *et al.:* Instantaneous blood flow in the human aorta. J. appl. Physiol. *20:* 691–695 (1965).

9 MORSE, R. L.: A mathematical model of the ballistocardiogram. Bibl. cardiol., vol. 19, pp. 136–140 (Karger, Basel 1967).

10 MASON, DEAN T.: Usefullness and limitations of the rate of rise of intraventricular pressure (dp/dt) in the evaluation of myocardial contractility in man. Amer. J. Cardiol. *23:* 516–527 (1969).

Author's address: D. M. AUSLANDER, Mechanical Engineering Department, University of California, *Berkeley, Calif.* (USA)

Proc. 16th ann. Meet. Ballistocard. Res. Soc., Atlantic City 1972;
Bibl. Cardiol. *32:* 22–25 (Karger, Basel 1973)

Simulation of the Contribution of the Heart to the Human Bcg

I. TOMEK

Department of Medicine, University of Alberta, Edmonton, Alberta

Introduction

In the past, there were several attempts to evaluate the contribution of the heart to the Bcg or to simulate the motion of the heart. One of them [1] is based on a simplified geometrical representation of the heart and experimentally obtained data about the volume of the ventricle, the motion of the heart and the atrial inflow. The resulting Bcg contribution obtained from this model is acceptable in that it agrees with results obtained by the same author on an analog of the rest of the circulation and combined with them gives Bcg wave forms comparable to those described in the literature. His model of the heart, however, unlike the rest of his model of the genesis of the Bcg is based on experimental data about the dynamical behavior of the heart and cannot be used to simulate the motion of the heart. Another model [2] of the heart is analytical; it only requires information about inflows and outflows and about the mechanical properties of the tissue surrounding the heart. This model, however, is overly simplified. It does not consider for example the changing shape of the heart and the changing distribution of mass in it, which is by far the most important factor causing the motion of the heart. Results obtained from this model are also unrealistic.

The model to be described here is analytical; it requires information about the mechanical properties of the thoracic cavity, inflows and outflows and changing volumes of ventricles and atria. Results obtained from it agree well with those obtained by NOORDERGRAAF which, although not a conclusive proof, is a strong indication of the validity of both models.

The Model

The heart is represented by two connected deformed hemispheres representing the atria and the ventricle – one hemisphere for both ventricles (blood + 250 cm^3 for muscle), one for both atria (blood + 50 cm^3 for muscle). Their shapes change with the continuously changing volumes and so does the position of the center of gravity of the whole. This representation is the basic part and contribution of this model. The heart is mechanically coupled to the rest of the thoracic cavity and is subjected to three kinds of forces:

(a) forces due to the changing relative position of the center of gravity of the heart;

(b) forces transmitted through the mechanical coupling to the rest of the thoracic cavity;

(c) forces due to inflows and outflows.

This physical model was converted into a set of nonlinear differential equations which were solved on a digital computer.

Results

Figures 1 and 2 show the input and output variables of a simulation. It can be seen that the results obtained are very similar to those published by NOORDERGRAAF [1]. There are differences in timing and to some extent in amplitudes. They are due to the fact that input values (volumes of ventricles and atria) used are different both in amplitude and in timing. They are almost identical, however, when one looks upon the physical causes of the major waves which are apparent from the comparison of the input and output data. This comparison shows that the three major waves are due to the atrial contraction, the isovolumic contraction of the ventricles and the beginning of filling of ventricles. Although the agreement of the two results is not a proof of validity of the two models since neither of them is irrefutably correct, it supports the conclusion that they are both good approximations to reality. In fact, one of them is based mostly on experimental data and makes simplification of a somewhat different nature than the other.

The model presented here has some advantages: It is more general and makes it possible to calculate data which have to be measured for (1). It is conceivable that this model could after some improvement be used for the simulation and analysis of the apex-cardiogram. Also it can be used to explain the physical meaning of some of the measured phenomena and the simulation of abnormal conditions.

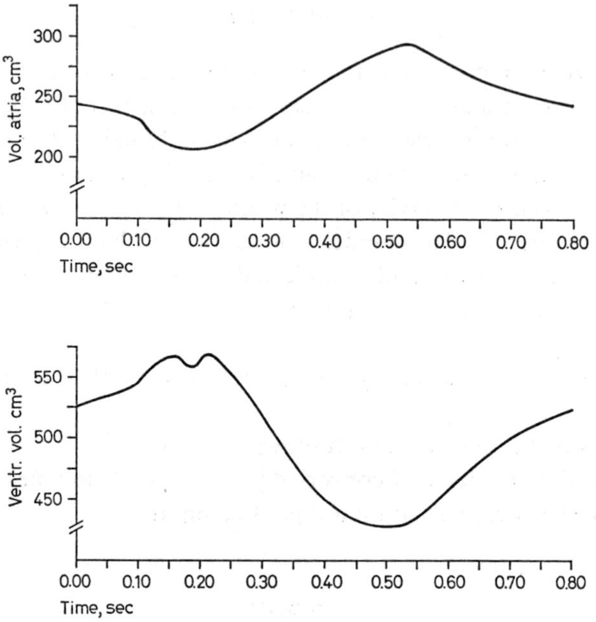

Fig. 1

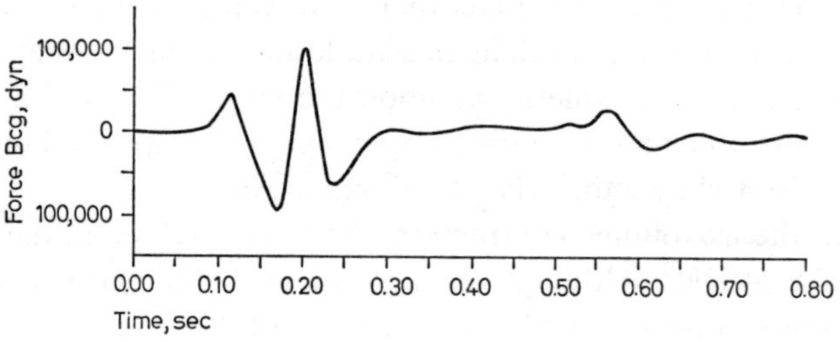

Fig. 2

Summary

This paper describes a simple model of the heart designed for the purpose of simulation of the motion of the heart and its contribution to the human Bcg. A preliminary result is presented.

Acknowledgement

This work was done during the tenure of a Fellowship of the Medical Research Council of Canada.

References

1 NOORDERGRAAF, A.: Further studies on a theory of the Bcg. Circulation *23:* 413 (1961).
2 HOOKS, L.E.: PhD. thesis, The Ohio State University (1970).

Author's address: Dr. IVAN TOMEK, Department of Medicine, University of Alberta, *Edmonton, Alberta* (Canada)

Proc. 16th ann. Meet. Ballistocard. Res. Soc., Atlantic City 1972;
Bibl. Cardiol. *32:* 26–36 (Karger, Basel 1973)

The Ballistocardiographic Relationship to the Hemodynamics of Valvular Aortic Stenosis[1]

D. H. JACKSON, MARJORIE TUCKER, W. H. BANCROFT, jr. and E. E. EDDLEMAN, jr.

Department of Medicine, University of Alabama School of Medicine and the Veterans Administration Hospital, Birmingham, Al.

Valvular aortic stenosis (VAS) is a common disorder in the population of the United States. It is difficult to evaluate clinically, often necessitating invasive catheterization study at a small but real risk to the patient. In children BARGERON [1] has shown that it is possible to use the ballistocardiogram (Bcg) to estimate whether the aortic valve gradient is greater than 35 mm Hg and, therefore, to assess the advisability of catheterization. There have been previous other studies of the relationship of the available Bcg data to the catheterization data in adults, but no studies have been published with such information utilizing the sophisticated computerized measurements of statistical relationships which are available at this time.

It was the purpose of this study to assess the available data in patients with pure VAS in order to define such relationships which may allow input of additional data into the initial or follow-up clinical evaluation of such patients without the necessity of invasive studies.

Materials and Methods

Subjects were those patients referred to the University of Alabama in Birmingham Hospital and the Veterans Administration Hospital in Birmingham. There were 23 patients, aged 16 to 74 years (mean 49.3), who had no cardiac disorder other than VAS by physical examination, history and cardiac catheterization. Five were female and 18 were male. None had evidence of myocardial infarction by history or by electrocardiogram (ECG). Two had no X-ray evidence of left ventricular enlargement but all others did. All had evidence of left ventricular hypertrophy by ECG voltage with or without additional standard

[1] Aided by USPH grants No. HE-11310 and 5 PO7 RR00145-09.

criteria. None were included who had arrhythmia, bundle branch block or intraventricular conduction defect. Time between Bcg and catheterization ranged from 24 h to 10 days, but 74% had both studies 48 h or less apart, and only four were studied 5 days or more apart.

Bcg's were recorded using an ultralow frequency air-bearing bed designed and built at the Johns Hopkins Medical School [2]. The bed had a natural frequency of 0.36 Hz and weighed 10.6 lb. with accelerometer and carotid transducer on it. A Northam Model A-14 accelerometer with a range of ± 0.5 g was mounted near the foot of the bed and measured head-foot acceleration. This transducer was connected to an Electronics for Medicine Model SGA-6 pressure amplifier in a DR-8 recorder. Each recording was preceded by a calibration consisting of the pressure steps from the pressure amplifier. These were periodically calibrated using an eccentric weight mounted on a synchronous motor fastened to the bed.

The held mid-expiration Bcg was recorded simultaneously with the Y-lead of the Frank vectorcardiogram and the carotid pressure pulse from a glycerine capsule transducer arrangement.

The records were measured by computer from magnetic tape recordings [3]. Durations, amplitudes and slopes measured from two to three complexes with the means, range and standard deviations are shown in table I. Terminology is standard, but in addition we

Table I. All Bcg measures from 23 patients with VAS

	N	Mean	Minimum	Maximum	Standard deviation
Amplitudes, cm/sec^2					
HI	23	2.038	0.533	5.463	1.191
I Maximum J	23	2.413	0.508	6.554	1.531
Maximum JK	23	2.228	0.787	5.034	1.283
HK	23	1.743	0.658	3.885	0.969
Durations, sec					
Q-H	23	0.102	0.062	0.134	0.022
Q-I	23	0.158	0.106	0.198	0.023
Q-Maximum J	23	0.233	0.138	0.306	0.049
Q-K	23	0.428	0.347	0.518	0.052
H-I	23	0.055	0.030	0.088	0.017
H-Maximum J	23	0.130	0.063	0.221	0.039
H-K	23	0.327	0.260	0.396	0.042
I-Maximum J	23	0.070	0.026	0.119	0.027
Slopes, cm/sec^2/sec					
H-I	23	−42.68	−8.62	−132.44	30.22
H-PI	23	−44.31	−7.18	−132.44	28.73
I-J	23	33.89	8.92	79.71	20.36
I-JP	23	44.83	8.16	100.10	27.01
HK/HI, ratio	23	0.941	0.629	1.525	0.304

have used the slope of the HI below the baseline (H-PI) and the slope of the IJ below the baseline (I-JP) (fig. 1). In addition, because some patients have more than one J peak, we have used the maximum J amplitude called Maximum J.

The record of the cardiac catheterization of each patient was analyzed by hand and various standard physical and hemodynamic values were computed. Aortic valve area was derived by standard methods using a mean valve gradient derived from the record by the method of visual comparison of areas [4].

Bcg classification was by a modification of the method of STARR and NOORDERGRAAF [5]. There were no full respiration cycle records available, but held inspiration and held expiration records were classified 1 through 4 separately and then together.

Statistical relationships were evaluated utilizing the computerized *Statistical Analysis System* which allows not only determination of simple correlations but additionally is capable of *Maximal R-Square Improvement* regression analysis [6]. Maximal R-Square Improvement is a technique which is almost as good as an all-possible analysis but much less computer time-consuming. It begins with the best single variable model with regard to R-square, then adds the best remaining variable for a two-variable model. It then pairs each of the two with every other variable not in the model to determine the effect of switching the two. Once all combinations have been tried, it then uses the one which improves the R-square the most. Having found the best two-variable model, the procedure adds a third variable and goes through the same process. The basic distinction between this technique and stepwise regression is that the latter always removes the worst and enters the best remaining variable, whereas Maximum R-Square Improvement checks on all combinations. It also allows one to force in for initial consideration such easily attainable items as age, sex, weight and height. Since some authors have suggested that these latter four items may significantly affect the Bcg, they were the first four to be considered by the program [7].

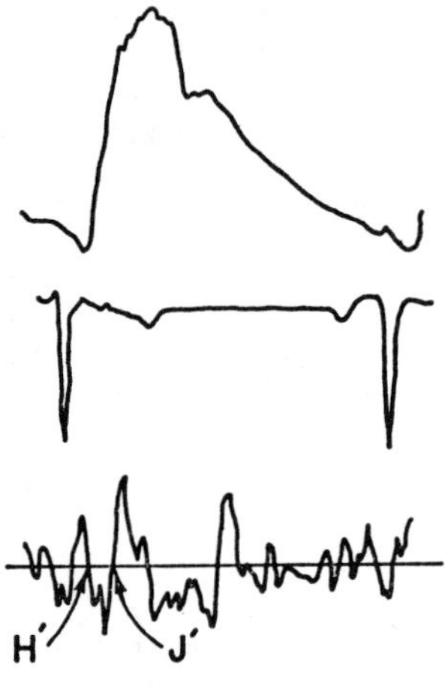

Fig. 1. Carotid pulse, VCG Y-lead, and ULF acceleration Bcg from top to bottom. H-PI slope and I-JP slope are the slope of H′ and J′, respectively, below the illustrated baseline.

Results

Ballistocardiographic measures are shown in table II. Data from a previously studied group of 200 healthy males, aged 42 to 54, are included for comparison. There are several measures which appear different in aortic stenosis.

Two patients were completely normal in all three conditions of respiration and combination of inspiratory and expiratory states. Four were class 4. The remainder were class 3.

Simple correlation of data revealed several strong relationships between hemodynamic measures and Bcg time intervals, amplitudes, slopes and ratios. These are not reported at this time, since other relationships are of more interest and are more precise.

Table II. Comparison of Bcg measures from VAS patients to a similarly aged group of healthy adult males

	Pensacola healthy males (age 42–54; n = 200) mean	Aortic stenosis (age 16–74; mean 49.3; n = 23) mean	AS versus normal
Amplitudes, cm/sec^2			
HI	2.5	2.038	lower
I Maximum J	3.6	2.413	lower
Maximum JK	3.3	2.228	lower
HK	2.2	1.743	lower
Durations, sec			
Q-H	0.09	0.102	longer
Q-I	0.16	0.158	same
Q-Maximum J	0.24	0.233	same
Q-K	0.36	0.428	longer
H-I	0.07	0.055	shorter
H-Maximum J	0.15	0.130	shorter
H-K	0.26	0.327	longer
I-Maximum J	0.08	0.070	shorter
Slopes, $cm/sec^2/sec$			
H-I	−37.9	−42.68	faster
H-PI	–	−44.31	
I-J	45.0	33.89	slower
I-JP	–	44.83	
HK/HI ratio	0.880	0.941	higher

Peak-to-peak aortic valve gradient (PPG) varied from 13 to 146 mm Hg (mean 69) in 23 patients (table III). It was apparent that 71% of the variance was explained by 10 Bcg-Physical-Historical (Bcg-PH) variables at 10° of freedom. Each of 12 variables contributed very highly significant data. Standard B values suggested that H-K duration and Q-K duration, representing mechanical and electromechanical ventricular ejection durations, were the most important variables by far.

Maximum aortic valve gradient (Max VG) varied from 22 to 173 mm Hg (mean 93) in 23 patients. Max R revealed that 55% of the variance was explained by seven Bcg-PH variables. In this one case, it is interesting to note that while at 10° of freedom level there is an R-square of 0.770, there are other statistical reasons for considering that to be an incorrectly strong correlation (table III). Of the parameters of significance, H-PI slope contributed most.

Mean aortic valve gradient (MVG) varied from 13 to 111 mm Hg (mean 57) in 23 patients. Max R analysis revealed that 79% of the variance is

Table III. VAS: statistical analysis result using *Maximal R-Square Improvement* regression analysis

Dependent variable	Probability > F at best improvement (degrees of freedom)	R-square at 10° of freedom	Coefficient of variation (%) at improvement (degrees of freedom)
Peak-to-peak valve gradient, mm Hg	0.0214 (8)	0.712	29.7 (8)
Maximum valve gradient, mm Hg	0.0932 (13)	0.770	36.5 (13)
Mean valve gradient, mm Hg	0.0356 (7)	0.788	26.3 (7)
Aortic valve area, cm^2	0.0003 (5)	0.747	4.54 (5)
Cardiac index, $l/min/m^2$	0.0012 (5)	0.891	4.68 (5)
Cardiac output, ml/min	0.0008 (5)	0.895	4.79 (5)
Effective stroke volume index/beat, $ml/beat/m^2$	0.0008 (5)	0.680	6.43 (5)
Aortic valve flow, ml/sec	0.0004 (5)	0.696	3.39 (5)
Aortic valve flow, ml/beat	0.0007 (5)	0.798	4.63 (5)

explained by 10 Bcg-PH variables (table III). A total of 13 such variables added highly significant contributions at 7° of freedom. Of these, the four amplitudes HI, HK, Max JK and I Max J, and H-K and Q-K durations are the most important as judged by Standard B values.

Cardiac index (CI) ranged from 1.87 to 4.63 (mean 2.97) l/min/m² in 20 patients. Max R revealed that 89% of the variance was explained by 7 Bcg-PH variables and that each of 12 such variables added very significant information at 5° of freedom (table III). Of these, I Max J amplitude and H-PI slope contributed the most information.

Cardiac output (CO) ranged from 3,590 to 9,954 (mean 5406) ml/min in 19 patients. 89% of the variance is explained by 6 Bcg-PH variables (tables III and IV). Very significant information is contributed by 11 variables (table V). Of these, H-PI slope and Max JK amplitude contribute the most individually.

Effective stroke volume index per beat (EVSVI) (ml/beat/m²) ranged from 7.9 to 59.3 (mean 37.2) in 16 patients. Max R analysis revealed that 68% of the variance was related to 4 Bcg-PH variables (table III). Highly significant contributions are made by 9 such variables. Of these, H-PI and I-JP slopes are the contributors of greatest significance.

Aortic valve flow (AVF) in ml/sec ranged from 154 to 424 (mean 249) in 17 patients. 70% of the variance is related to 4 Bcg-PH variables (table III).

Table IV. Maximum R-square improvement for dependent variable COCCMIN at 10° of freedom

Source	DF	Prob > F	R-square
Regression	6	0.0005	0.89454731
Error	10		
Corrected total	16		

Source	Prob > T	STD B values
Mean		
Weight	0.0003	0.80195837
HR	0.0042	−0.39786300
IMAXJDUR	0.0003	0.87751322
Height	0.0033	−0.70484850
Q–IDUR	0.0135	0.34196664
HK–HIRAT	0.0244	−0.34168745

COCCMIN = Cardiac output in cc/min; HR = heart rate; IMAXJDUR = I-Maximum J peak duration; Q-IDUR = Q-I duration; HK-HIRAT = HK/HI ratio.

Highly significant contributions are made by 9 variables. Of these, H-I and H-PI slopes were the largest contributors by far.

Aortic valve flow in ml/beat (AVF/beat) ranged from 38 to 117 (mean 72.4) in 18 patients. 80% of the variance was related to 6 Bcg-PH variables (table III). Highly significant components are contributed by 11 variables. Of these, Q-H and H-Max J durations are the major contributors.

Aortic valve area (AVA) cm^2 ranged from 0.438 to 1.682 (mean 0.799) in 17 patients. Max R revealed that 75% of the variance is related to 4 Bcg-PH variables (table III). Nine variables are contributors of significance concerning variance of this dependent measure. Of these, HK/HI ratio and H-Max J duration are the most important variables.

These Maximum R-Square results may be utilized in producing regression equations for prediction of the dependent variables, such as cardiac index in patients with pure aortic stenosis. This was attempted for all of the previously mentioned variables (table VI). When the equations are used to predict these variables for the group whose data were used to derive the equation, it is evident that the predicted value and the individual directly measured variable

Table V. Maximum R-square improvement for dependent variable COCCMIN at best improvement (5° of freedom)

Source	DF	Prob > F	R-square
Regression	11	0.0008	0.99163451
Error	5		
Corrected total	16		
Source		**Prob > T**	**STD B values**
Mean			
Q-KDUR		0.0011	0.87434468
Weight		0.0095	0.49538157
HPI Slope		0.0010	−1.75076644
H-ISLOPE		0.0013	1.16006828
Q-IDUR		0.0065	0.35667473
Height		0.0004	−1.08596786
IMAXJDUR		0.0007	1.36028204
Age		0.0009	0.74984657
MAXJKAMP		0.0023	−1.72267260
Hkamp		0.0073	0.97837305
IJP Slope		0.0766	0.30276105

COCCMIN = *Cardiac output* in cc/min; Q-KDUR, IMAXJDUR, and Q-IDUR = duration of each; AMP = amplitude. HPI Slope and IJP Slope are as illustrated in figure 1.

Table VI. Prediction of valve area (cm^2) compared to catheterization computation of area

	Observed value	Predicted value
Original patients with AS	0.770	0.961
	0.650	0.515
	1.250	1.144
	0.593	0.742
	0.706	0.728
	0.475	0.685
	0.438	0.366
	0.852	0.623
	0.694	0.849
	0.637	0.741
	1.136	0.929
	1.355	1.346
	0.537	0.381
	1.682	1.452
	0.616	0.723
	0.530	0.475
	0.670	0.933
New Patients with AS (not used to formulate regression equation)	1.160	0.362
	0.720	0.819
	1.210	1.446
	2.700	1.709
	2.280	0.640
	1.120	0.369
	1.420	0.551
	1.060	1.225

Table VII. Maximum R-square improvement for dependent variable VALVEAR at 10° of freedom

Source	DF	Prob > F	R-square
Regression	4	0.0053	0.74701626
Error	10		
Corrected total	14		
Source		**Prob > T**	**STD B values**
Mean			
Q-HDUR		0.0012	0.89576432
HK-HIRAT		0.0030	−0.72134255
Sex		0.0029	−0.76355552
H-MXJDUR		0.0933	−0.32610515

VALVEAR = Valve area; DUR = duration; RAT = ratio; MX = maximum.

Table VIII. Maximum R-square improvement for dependent variable REPAREA (valve Area with additional patients added to first group at 10° of freedom)

Source	DF	Prob > F	R-square
Regression	12	0.0010	0.91841301
Error	10		
Corrected total	22		
Source		**Prob > T**	**STD B values**
Mean			
Age		0.0151	−0.42385195
HK-HIRAT		0.0003	−0.99801264
HPI Slope		0.0100	1.30198085
H-I Slope		0.0004	−2.20062446
Q-IDUR		0.0001	2.33360091
IMAXJDUR		0.0001	3.63981154
Q-MXJDUR		0.0001	−3.43461359
IMAXJAMP		0.0043	−2.79048389
HIAMP		0.0141	1.45137226
Sex		0.0235	−0.30288236
Q-KDUR		0.0322	−0.30777832
MAXJKAMP		0.0956	0.75465986

Improved R-square is evident (0.91841301) (see table VII). AMP = Amplitude; RAT = ratio; DUR = duration; HPI Slope as in figure 1.

are reasonably close. However, when prediction of the dependent variables is attempted for each of a smaller additional group of individuals with aortic stenosis, it is evident that in some cases the resultant is very close to the actually measured variable, but in others it was extremely different (table VI).

Additionally, when a larger number of subjects is added to the Maximum R-square data bank, the resultant R-square at 10° of freedom was usually better than when the smaller original group was utilized to produce most of the data previously presented (tables VII and VIII).

Discussion

Our results indicate that there are substantial differences in some durations, amplitudes and slopes in VAS when compared to healthy normals. Additionally, there are numerous moderately strong correlations of Bcg variables with direct invasive measures.

Of more importance, statistical study suggests that there are within the ultralow frequency Bcg waveform items which when combined will surely allow prediction of hemodynamic measures. It is quite evident, however, that when such derived prediction equations are used for individuals, they break down currently. The reasons include probably some which are not evident at this time but the data suggest that they will be shown to include a need for much larger groups of invasively studied patients with Bcg data. Since there appears to be much larger beat-to-beat variation in these measures from the Bcg than has been previously reported, subsequent studies will require data acquisition from larger numbers of complexes than were utilized here, perhaps using some type of averaging.

It is possible to computerize the Bcg and analyze it without hand measuring. However, it is not yet possible to accurately predict these hemodynamic variables from such ballistocardiographic measurements though it seems certain that it will be possible in the near future.

Summary

(1) There are clear differences in some Bcg measures in aortic stenosis when compared to measures from healthy individuals.

(2) There are numerous strong correlations between individual Bcg measures and hemodynamic measures.

(3) *Maximum R-square* analysis reveals that there are moderate to very strong indications that certain hemodynamic variables are reflected in the Bcg.

(4) R-square is improved by adding larger numbers of patients to the basic group.

(5) It is not yet possible to predict individual hemodynamic variables with acceptable accuracy, but with larger numbers of subjects and utilizing more complexes for analysis it clearly seems possible in the near future.

References

1 Bargeron, L. M.: The force ballistocardiogram as an index of severity in congenital aortic stenosis. Circulation *37:* 238–243 (1968).

2 Harrison, W. K. and Talbot, S. A.: Two new forms of ultra-low frequency ballistocardiograph. Bibl. cardiol., Vol. 19, pp. 13–18 (Karger, Basel 1967).

3 Bancroft, W.H., jr.; Tucker, M.; Jackson, D.H., and Eddelman, E.E., jr.: Automatic processing of ballistocardiograms by computer. Bibl. Cardiol. (in press).

4 Potanin, C.; Jackson, D.H., and Burdeshaw, J.: Determination of valvular pressure gradients by visual comparison of area. J. appl. Physiol. *29:* 717–719 (1970).

5 STARR, I. and NOORDERGRAAF, A.: Ballistocardiography in cardiovascular research (Lippincott, Philadelphia 1967).
6 BARR, A.J. and GOODNIGHT, J.H.: Statistical analysis system (Department of Statistics, North Carolina State University, Raleigh, N.C., December 1971).
7 JACKSON, D.H.; OBERMAN, A.; MITCHELL, R.E., and GRAYBIEL, A.: Factors contributing to the ballistocardiographic waveform in healthy middle-aged males. Amer. J.Cardiol. *20:* 531–540 (1967).

Author's address: Prof.Dr. DAVID H.JACKSON, Department of Medicine, University of Alabama School of Medicine, *Birmingham, Ala.* (USA)

Proc. 16th ann. Meet. Ballistocard. Res. Soc., Atlantic City 1972;
Bibl. Cardiol. *32:* 37–41 (Karger, Basel 1973)

Cardiac Weakness and Incoordination in a Large Population of Ambulatory Cardiac Patients[1]

I. STARR

Department of Therapeutic Research, School of Medicine,
University of Pennsylvania, Philadelphia, Pa.

Studies on an electrical model of the circulation by VERDOUW [1] have given us renewed confidence in our ability to interpret clinical records of the carotid pulse derivative (CPD) and the ULF force ballistocardiogram (Bcg) in physiological terms. The magnitude of measurements such as the maximum amplitude of the carotid pulse derivative (PD max); the overall amplitude, the depth of the I wave, and the slope of the HI segment of the Bcg are plainly related to various aspects of the strength of the cardiac contraction [2]. Also, abnormalities of contour of these records can easily be produced in models by simulating an irregular cardiac ejection curve, so, when similar abnormalities are seen in the clinic, they are to be attributed to an irregular or incoordinate cardiac contraction [1].

Encouraged by the new data, so largely confirmatory of previous views [2], I have reviewed the clinical records taken over the last three years to ascertain the relative frequency of weakness and incoordination in ambulatory cardiac cases. A preliminary report has been made [3].

Subjects and Methods

Table I gives the cardiac diagnosis of the 1,048 cases where records were reviewed for this study. All were ambulatory. No patient in the acute stages of cardiac infarction or congestive failure was included in the series.

The CPD and Bcg were taken after a 15-min rest period with the patient recumbent.

[1] This work was supported by USPHS grant HE 625 CVB.

Results

All the records had been read by me the day they were taken, and my opinion of their normality or abnormality was recorded at that time. When reading the Bcg, judgment of cardiac strength was based on overall amplitude of the Bcg, the depth of the I wave, and the slope of the HI segment [2], which were not measured if they were normal to inspection. The diagnosis of cardiac incoordination was based on irregularities of contours as described [2]. When reading the pulse derivative such judgments were based on the amplitude of PD max and the presence of abnormalities of the contour, as has also been

Table I. Primary cardiac diagnosis of 1,048 patients tested by carotid pulse derivative and force Bcg, since 1964

Coronary heart disease	26%
No heart disease	19%
Hypertensive heart disease	16%
Rheumatic heart disease	7%
Congenital heart disease	3%
Hyperthyroid	2%
Arteriosclerotic heart disease	2%
Pericarditis	1%
Other types of heart disease	7%
No heart disease diagnosed by conventional methods, but our tests indicated myocardial abnormality	17%

Table II. Cardiac weakness and incoordination in over 1,000 ambulatory cases

	As judged by PD	As judged by Bcg
Weakness without incoordination	< 2%	< 2%
Incoordination without weakness	42%	29%

Table III. Relation of contour abnormalities of the PD to those of the Bcg in 1,035 cases in which both records were satisfactory

Carotid PD and Bcg, both normal	38%
Carotid PD and Bcg, both abnormal	43%
Carotid PD normal, Bcg abnormal	19%
Carotid PD abnormal, Bcg normal	< 1%

described [4]. From this inspection of the records, table II was compiled. Table III shows the relation of the contour abnormalities of the two records to one another in this same series of patients.

Discussion

The results recorded in table II show clearly that when reading these records I have been diagnosing cardiac incoordination in these patients far more frequently than I have been diagnosing weakness. But several difficulties should be discussed. By measuring certain aspects of these records our judgment of cardiac weakness can easily be made quantitative, but for the diagnosis of incoordination we must rely on differences of contour that cannot be easily expressed quantitatively. And where it is best to put the dividing line between normal and abnormal cardiac function is still uncertain.

Despite such difficulties more strictly quantitative studies have yielded similar results. For example, STARR and OGAWA [4] worked out the normal scatter of PD max in the pulses from the *brachial artery* of healthy persons. In these subjects, PD max was significantly correlated with age. One hundred ward patients, most of them cardiacs, were then tested. When the lower normal limits were defined as 2σ below the regression, not one subnormal case was found.

More recently, normal standards for the *carotid* PD max were set up from tests made on 50 healthy persons. In them also PD max was significantly correlated with age, the regression being:

$$\text{PD max mm Hg/sec} = -5.9 \text{ age years} + 986.$$

Using the convential 2σ below the regression as our lower normal limit, only 3 out of over 1,000 patients were found below this limit.

In early work with the Bcg overall amplitude the vertical I–J distance was used as an index of strength [4]. Statistical standards were set up over 20 years ago, but they were never used extensively in clinical work, largely because, when the lower limit of normal was set as 2σ below the mean, the cases thus identified as having significantly weak hearts were so few.

Obviously, therefore, by using quantitative methods which seem well based physiologically, and which clearly demonstrate cardiac weakness in a few patients, we find evidence that the heart is weak very rarely, although hundreds of ambulatory cases with strong clinical evidence of advanced heart disease have been tested.

In contrast, our qualitative methods demonstrate incoordination of the cardiac contraction in literally hundreds of ambulatory cases, and the known errors inherent in recording the pulse [5] suggest that we may fail to demonstrate this abnormality in many cases in which it is present. So there is a striking contrast between the frequency of myocardial incoordination and the rarity of cardiac weakness in our ambulatory cases of cardiac disease, and these findings drive me to a new conception of the downward course of chronic heart disease.

The animal experiments of the physiologists and pharmacologists have led to the belief that, when the myocardium of any patient fails, it fails as a whole. That this is true in acute animal experiments no one doubts, and when the patient is in extremis such generalized failure undoubtedly occurs also. But earlier in the course of chronic cardiac illness such generalized failure is rarely encountered. In the downward progress of cardiac disease incoordination is commonly detected long before weakness, so we must believe that one or more parts of the myocardium usually fail first, while other parts are still contracting normally. Indeed, it seems likely that the more normal parts of the heart, by contracting more strongly, compensate for the weakness of the weaker parts; as disease progresses, more and more parts of the myocardium become abnormal until weakness of the whole heart manifests itself.

This theory is supported not only by our findings, but also by the usual pathological anatomy of coronary heart disease, some vessels being narrowed or blocked when others remain normally patent.

To this theory there is an important corollary. Those seeking to identify myocardial abnormality early in the course of heart disease should seek evidence of the incoordination of the cardiac contraction rather than of its weakness.

Conclusions

In a series of over 1,000 cardiac cases, studied by taking simultaneous records of the carotid pulse derivative and the ULF force ballistocardiogram, incoordination of the cardiac contraction was diagnosed frequently, weakness of the heart very rarely. The findings indicate that the myocardium usually fails, not as a whole, but bit by bit. In the early stages of myocardial disease the normal parts of the heart compensate for the abnormal by contracting more strongly, so incoordination manifests itself long before weakness of the heart as a whole.

Summary

Simultaneous records of the force Bcg and carotid pulse derivative have been taken routinely at the University Hospital since 1964, chiefly on ambulatory cardiac patients. Those taken during the last three years, numbering over 1,000, have recently been analyzed to find the relative frequency of the two chief manifestations of physiological abnormality found in both the heart and other muscles, weakness and incoordination. Judged both by the PD and the Bcg, weakness without incoordination is rare in the group, while incoordination without other evidence of weakness is very common, about 40%. Another 40% show evidence of both incoordination and weakness. We concluded that, as a rule, incoordination precedes weakness in the downward progression of myocardial disease.

In chronic heart disease, the heart usually fails, not as a whole, as in the acute experiments of the physiologists, but piece by piece, a finding in complete accord with the usual pathological anatomy of coronary artery disease. To detect myocardial disease early, one should seek for evidence of cardiac incoordination rather than weakness.

References

1 Verdouw, P.D.: Ballistics of ventricular performance; diss. biomed. engineer., University of Pennsylvania (1970).

2 Starr, I. and Noordergraaf, A.: Ballistocardiography in cardiovascular research (North Holland, Amsterdam/Lippincott, Philadelphia 1967).

3 Starr, I.; Noordergraaf, A., and Verdouw, P.D.: A new theory on the course of development of myocardial disease. Clin. Res. *19:* 559 (1971). (abstract)

4 Starr, I. and Ogawa, S.: A clinical study of the 1st derivative of the brachial pulse. Normal standards and abnormalities encountered in heart disease. Amer. Heart J. *64:* 482 (1963).

5 Starr, I.: Quantitative studies on the errors of the pulse, when used to estimate cardiac function. Amer. Heart J. *77:* 222 (1969).

Author's address: Isaac Starr, M.D., 851 Gates Memorial Pavilion, Hospital of the University of Pennsylvania, 3600 Spruce Street, *Philadelphia, PA 19174* (USA)

Proc. 16th ann. Meet. Ballistocard. Res. Soc., Atlantic City 1972;
Bibl. Cardiol. *32:* 42–44 (Karger, Basel 1973)

Cardiac Function during Cheyne-Stokes Respiration[1]

I. Starr

Department of Therapeutic Research, School of Medicine, University of Pennsylvania, Philadelphia, Pa.

Cheyne-Stokes respiration is a type of periodic breathing seen frequently in sick cardiacs and in patients with cerebral abnormalities. It is also seen in healthy persons at high altitude, or when breathing gas mixtures low in oxygen. Typically, breathing is interrupted by periods of apnoea, after which respiration begins feebly, slowly increases, to a maximum which is often abnormally vigorous, then slowly subsiding until another apnoea supervenes. The length of the cycles, and of the apnoeic periods, varies.

Among the large numbers of cardiac patients tested in my laboratory during the last few years, there has been opportunity to secure ULF force Bcg's on seven who exhibited Cheyne-Stokes respiration, and the findings in all were so similar that a single example will suffice.

Figure 1 shows the typical result. During the period of apnoea the Bcg is normal or nearly so, while the patient is overbreathing this record is found to have deteriorated.

At first thought this finding seemed strange and unexpected. I had supposed that these abnormal hearts would beat best when they were well supplied with oxygen, worst when the supply was low. Certainly blood would be better oxygenated when breathing was vigorous than during apnoea. Our results are contrary to such expectations.

Careful studies in other laboratories have given us other facts to keep in mind. A slow circulation time is found in patients showing Cheyne-Stokes respiration [1, 2]. In normal dogs, when lung-to-brain circulation time was increased experimentally, Cheyne-Stokes breathing followed [3]. Also the

[1] This work was supported by USPHS grant HE 625 CVB.

arterial blood gas tension of O_2 and CO_2 does not fluctuate pari-passu with the changes of breathing, there is considerable phase shift [1].

Obviously, the delay in blood reaching the respiratory center could account for the lag in the respiratory response to change in blood gas content. But whether this delay could account for the cardiac changes seen in Cheyne-Stokes breathing I doubt; the coronary circulation is so much closer to the lungs than is the brain, and in our cases the Bcg still looks normal at the end of long periods of apnoea.

Obviously, much more work needs to be done to interpret our findings, but we clearly have a fact to add to the knowledge of Cheyne-Stokes respiration. A marked variation in cardiac function is part of this cyclical phenomenon; as far as I know, this has not been reported before.

One wonders if the cardiac difficulties could be primary; in Cheyne-Stokes breathing, when cardiac function is at its worst, hyperventilation is at its greatest; every clinician expects poor cardiac function to cause hyperventilation. This 'cardiac' theory leads to the expection that overbreathing would cease when the heart beats more normally, as it does in our cases.

But one can also think of the cardiac effect as secondary. That lack of oxygen stimulates the myocardium is well known [4]. Bad hearts can be stimulated as well as good ones, and stimulation makes many bad hearts beat more normally. What we see in the Cheyne-Stokes respiration might be the

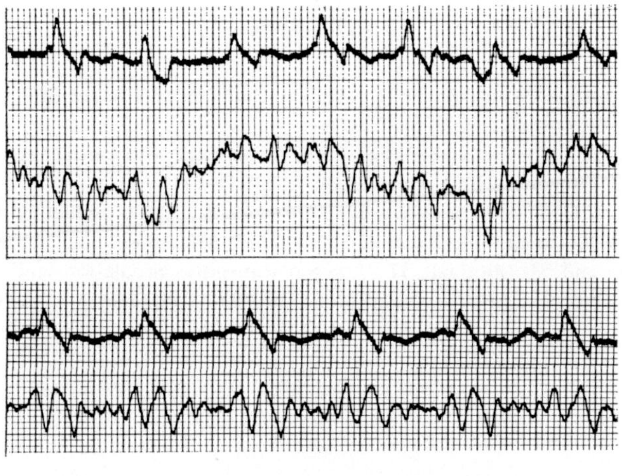

Fig. 1. Cardiac function in Cheyne-Stokes respiration. Carotid pulse derivative over ULF force Bcg, during hyperventilation (top), and during apnoea (bottom). Records of F. R., age 51, former cardiac infarction, BP 120/95. Note Bcg improvement during apnoea.

result of periodic cardiac stimulation from anoxemia. To learn how this stimulation fits in with the other findings in this fascinating cyclic phenomenon would require much more study than I have time to make. I mention these few cases in the hope of tempting someone into the field, for the Bcg is well qualified to aid in the solution of problems of this kind.

Conclusion

Marked cyclical variation in cardiac function accompanies Cheyne-Stokes respiration. The heart beat is strongest and best coordinated during the apnoeic period.

Summary

Over the years an occasional sick cardiac tested on the Bcg has proved to have Cheyne-Stokes respiration, and records have been taken both during breathing and during apnoea. The findings in all these patients were similar, and they were the reverse of my expectations. The heart beats much more strongly and with better coordination during the periods of apnoea than during breathing. Apparently, the increasing anoxemia of the apnoeic periods stimulates the abnormal heart as it does the normal heart, when healthy persons breath gas mixtures low in oxygen content.

References

1 LANGE, R.L. and HECHT, H.H.: The mechanism of Cheyne-Stokes respiration. J.clin.Invest. *41:* 42 (1962).
2 PRYN, W.W.: Cheyne-Stokes respiration in patients with cardiac enlargement and prolonged circulation time. Circulation *4:* 233 (1951).
3 GUYTON, A.C.; CROWELL, J.W., and MOORE, J.W.: Basic oscillating mechanism of Cheyne-Stokes breathing. Amer.J.Physiol. *187:* 395 (1956).
4 STARR, I. and MCMICHAEL, H.: Oxygen transport, circulation and respiration in healthy subjects at stimulated altitudes of 16,000–18,000 feet. J.appl.Physiol. *1:* 430 (1948).

Author's address: ISAAC STARR, M.D., 851 Gates Memorial Pavilion, Hospital of the University of Pennsylvania, 3600 Spruce Street, *Philadelphia, PA 19174* (USA)

Proc. 16th ann. Meet. Ballistocard. Res. Soc., Atlantic City 1972;
Bibl. Cardiol. *32:* 45–49 (Karger, Basel 1973)

Ballistocardiographic Changes with A–V Fistula Formation

D. C. Fischer

Good Samaritian Hospital and College of Medicine,
University of Cincinnati, Cincinnati, Ohio

Introduction

The opportunity to study ballistocardiographic findings in patients with arteriovenous (A-V) fistulae is very limited. The largest series reported was studied between 1943 and 1946 at the Military Vascular Surgery Center at Ashford General Hospital by Elkins and Warren [1]. Forty-seven of their patients with traumatic A-V fistulae had a ballistocardiogram (Bcg) as part of an evaluation of cardiac output. It is unfortunate, in a very limited sense, that such cases are rare in civilian medicine because the attendant pathophysiology represents an exceptional clinical situation in which to study the effect of certain cardiovascular (C-V) changes on the Bcg.

An unusual opportunity to study such cases has been available to us during the past 10 years. A group of children was subjected to the surgical establishment of a large A-V fistula in an attempt to cause overgrowth of a leg retarded by poliomyelitis. The procedure was suggested by the observation that traumatic A-V fistulae sometimes result in enlargement of the extremity distally [2]. The overall outcome of this program is not the subject of this paper. Rather, this report deals with the ballistocardiographic findings in these children before and during the course of the A-V fistula.

Clinical Material

Nineteen children, ranging in age from 7 to 13 years, had either a mid-femoral or popliteal A-V fistula created. The size of the fistulae ranged from 1.7 to 2.3 cm along the length of the vessels, hence can all be considered to be hemodynamically significant. Without exception, all patients clinically had normal C-V systems prior to creation of the fistulae, and specifically, their Bcg's were all normal[1].

The duration of the maintenance of the fistulae to date has averaged 5 years. At appropriate periods during this time, the C-V system of each child has been re-evaluated, at times including repeat Bcg. No patient has developed significant clinical problems of any kind. A more detailed study of the Bcg's has been completed on four of our patients. This study is the primary purpose of this communication.

[1] All tracings were recorded on an air-bearing, ultra-low frequency machine. Manufacturer: Royal Medical Corporation, Huntsville, Ala.

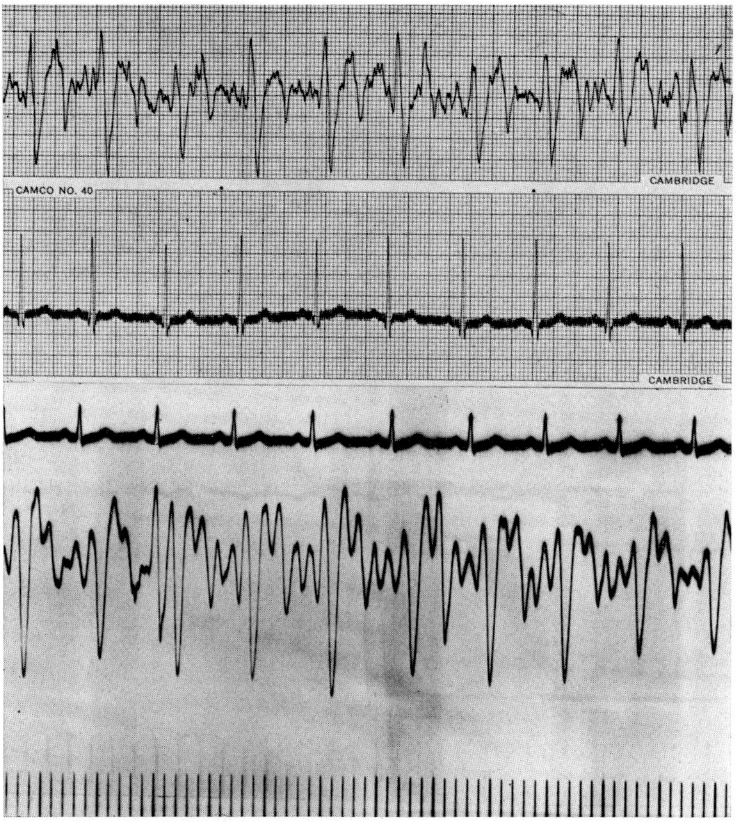

Fig. 1. Patient A.D.: tracings recorded just prior to (above) and 8 years after (below) the creation of an A-V fistula while it was still functioning.

Results

Patient J.A. was 13 years old when the fistula was created and it was maintained for 49 months. Two significant Bcg changes occurred. First there was a definite increase in the segment lengths throughout. Secondly, no change occurred in the timing of the H-I-J-K portion, but the L-M-N portion of the Bcg was seriously delayed in timing. A Bcg taken one year after closure revealed a return of all phases to pre-fistula levels.

Patient A.D., actually the first patient operated, was 8 years old when the fistula was formed and it was maintained for 8 years. Again, there was marked increase in the segment lengths, and again (the finding we feel is of special interest), there was no change in the timing of the H-I-J-K portion and considerable delay in the diastolic section of the trace (fig. 1). Again, a Bcg done 16 months after closure of the fistula showed a return of the segment lengths and timings to pre-fistula levels.

The third patient, M.L., had his fistula from age 12 to 16, a total of 52 months. The segment length increase was similar to the others. In this patient, there was only slight increase in the overall timing of the diastolic portion. The K-L segment timing was increased 50% in duration, but the N point appeared to be somewhat shortened, which accounted for the overall appearance of minimal increase.

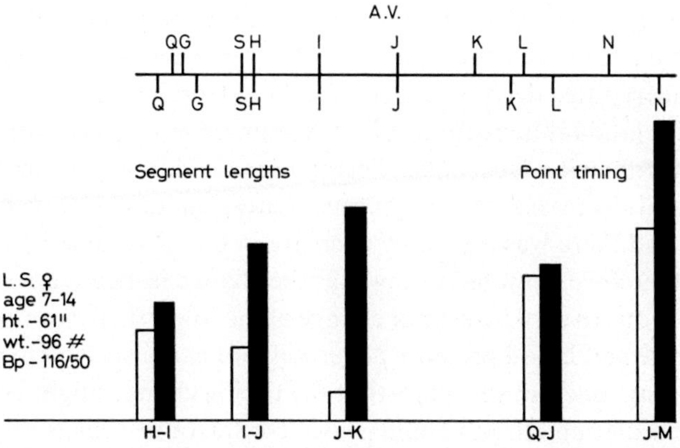

Fig. 2. Patient L.S.: timing of Bcg and ECG points are plotted for the recording before the fistula was present (above the line) and for the tracing taken while the fistula was functioning 7 years later (below the line). In the plots of segment lengths and point timings, the first column is from before the fistula and the second from the tracing 7 years later.

Finally, patient L.S. is one of the patients who still has the fistula functioning. She was 7 years old when it was created; she is now 14. Her Bcg also shows the increased segment lengths, a distinct prolongation of the diastolic timing, and no change in the timing of the ejection fraction (fig. 2). Upon acute occlusion with a cuff, the segment lengths decreased mildly but the timing changes remained.

Discussion

It is reasonable to assume that any ballistocardiographic change that developed in these children after the fistulae were present was the direct result of the pathophysiology of the fistula and not due to any coincident cardiac or vascular disease, in view of their age and general good health. Consequently, the changes one might expect would be those due to decreased peripheral resistance, increased total blood volume, or increased cardiac output singly or combined. It is well established that these are the abnormalities found in such patients as long as congestive heart failure does not supervene. The increase in segment lengths found here is in agreement with the findings of ELKINS and WARREN [1] 25 years ago, and KLENSCH *et al.* [3] and others since. The timing delay in the latter portion of the tracings, however, has not been noted to our knowledge, and is consistent in these patients.

HOLMAN [4] made the most comprehensive review of the pathophysiology of A-V fistula. He noted the following changes when a fistula was created: increased heart rate, decreased diastolic blood pressure, increased cardiac output and a gradual increase in blood volume. On occlusion of the fistula, he found the following *immediate* effects: increased blood pressure, decreased pulse rate and decreased cardiac output. Later, the blood pressure returned to normal, and there was a *gradual* decrease in blood volume and pulse rate.

One is, therefore, tempted to say that the change in Bcg segment length in A-V fistula is due to cardiac output change alone, since there is ample evidence that heart rate and blood pressure *per se* will not cause such a change. By the same reasoning, one can speculate that the timing change might be due to the change in circulating blood volume, since considerable time is required after closure of the fistula before it returns to normal.

One finding of VERDOUW [5] using the pulsatile flow analog model may be of some interest in regard to these changes. He found that the timing of the L wave was not affected by change in peripheral resistance.

Summary and Conclusion

We have found in a series of four patients that a large surgically constructed A-V fistula causes an increase in the length of most segments of the Bcg, probably best relatable to increased cardiac output. This agrees essentially with the findings of others who have reported. We found, further, that the timing of the later, diastolic, waves was delayed and that this delay subsides only after the fistula is no longer present for some period of time. Since peripheral resistance and cardiac output change immediately upon occlusion of the fistula, these would appear *not* to be the cause of these timing delays. The increase in blood volume seems to be the best tentative explanation for them.

References

1 Elkins, D.C. and Warren, J.V.: Arteriovenous fistulas. J.amer.med.Ass. *134:* 1524–1528 (1947).

2 Janes, J.M. and Jennings, W.K.: Effect of induced arteriovenous fistula on leg length: 10-year observations. Proc. Staff Mtg., Mayo Clin. *36:* 1 (1961).

3 Klensch, H.; Hohnen, H.W. und Richter, W.: Das Schlagvolumen des Herzens vor und nach Operation traumatischer arteriovenöser Fisteln der unteren Extremitäten. Z.KreislForsch. *48:* 153 (1959).

4 Holman, E.: Abnormal arteriovenous communications: peripheral and intracardiac, acquired and congenital; 2nd ed. (Thomas, Springfield 1968).

5 Verdouw, P.D.: Ballistics of ventricular performance (University Microfilms, Ann Arbor 1970).

Author's address: Donald C. Fischer, M.D., Good Samaritian Hospital, 3217 Clifton Avenue, *Cincinnati, OH 45220* (USA)

Proc. 16th ann. Meet. Ballistocard. Res. Soc., Atlantic City 1972;
Bibl. Cardiol. *32:* 50–57 (Karger, Basel 1973)

Effects of Hypertension on High-Frequency (Acceleration) direct Body Ballistocardiography

N. J. WINER

Lenox Hill Hospital, New York City, N.Y.

Several recent reports relative to the ULF Bcg – in one, as an incidental remark [6]; in another, as a primary clinical study [16] with suggested corroboration by the analogue computer [17] appeared to indicate that hypertension has no effect on the form of the Bcg. Studies with the high-frequency (acceleration) direct body ballistocardiograph (HF [a] DB Bcg) are presented here to question this suggestion.

Physiologic observations on the hypertensive effects on cardiac function have established: *hemodynamically*, an inverse relation between peripheral vascular resistance and cardiac output and index [12, 13]; an increase in end diastolic pressure by vasopressor infusion [8]; an increase in stroke volume by increasing aortic pressure with end diastolic volume constant [9]; impedance as a determinant of stroke work [14] and velocity of myocardial fiber shortening [18]; an increase in peak dp/dt [5, 19] particularly with increased muscle mass [15] and the degree of this increase, as well as, tension, dT/dt and, under certain circumstances, isovolumetric period and preejection period/left ventricular ejection time (PEP/LVET) [20] determined by the arterial diastolic pressure [2, 7, 19]; *metabolically*, with pressure work reflected by tension time index, accentuation of the greater oxygen and substrate requirement of pressure over flow work [4, 10]. In the face of these, some alterations in the form of the Bcg might well be expected.

[1] This study was aided by a grant from the Florence G. Heller Foundation and, in part, by the Xerox Corporation, Bertram Hoffberger and the family of Mr. SAMUEL W. HUROWITZ.

Method

The physical characteristics of the HF (a) DB Bcg [1, 3], the nature of its record and application [21, 33] have been previously described and will not be repeated in the interests of space. Add to these only the recently proposed 'rule of H-J_R[2] reciprocity' [23]: both of these segments appear contained in the corresponding upstroke of the carotid pulse, with J_R accentuation proposed as compensatory to antecedent HI deterioration (early 'H'). Recordings were made both on a Sanborn Twin-Beam standardized against a beam displacement of 1 cm by 1 mV for overall dynamic perspective and serial comparison and

[2] J_R and J_L notations are retained as proposed by the Committee on Nomenclature [11] but not intended to represent right and left ventricular contractions.

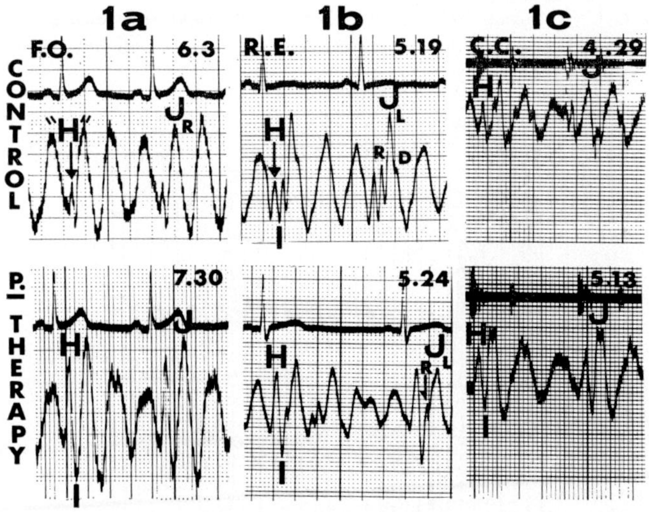

Fig. 1a. F.O. Age 24. Male. 6.3.69: BP 182/120. Note early diminished 'H' with a $q_{(Ecg)}$-'H' interval of 0.09–0.1 sec and accentuation of J_R (rule of H-J_R reciprocity). 7.30.69 (following 5 days of bed rest without medication): BP 154/100. HIJ is restored to an essentially normal pattern with $q_{(Ecg)}$-H now a normal 0.16 sec while J_R is submerged in the trough of HIJ.

Fig. 1b. R.E. Age 29. Male. 5.19.71: BP 202/104. Note diminished, slightly early, H ($q_{(Ecg)}$-H of 0.12 sec) with slight accentuation of J_R. 5.24.71 (following simple tranquilization therapy): BP 138/86. HIJ is restored to normal with a $q_{(Ecg)}$-H interval of 0.16 sec while J_R remains a small notch on the ascending limb to the J_R peak.

Fig. 1c. C.C. Age 46. Male. 4.29.59 (2 days post convulsive seizure): BP 164/120. All pattern segments are diminished. 5.13.59 (following PETN and Rauwiloid® therapy). BP 152/104. Amplitude of all segments is improved with apparently normal configuration.

an Electronics for Medicine DR 8 for correlation of different parameters and qualitative segmental characterization. The studies are based on the intervention method with the patient serving as his own control.

Studies

Case I. F.O. A 24-year-old male with known hypertension for several years established as 'essential' by renal arteriographic and chemical studies: BP 182/120. Bcg: reduced amplitude with early 'H' followed by accentuated J_R which persisted despite various types of antipressor drug therapy. Following five days of hospitalization at bed rest without medication: BP 152/100. Bcg: amplitude is restored with 'normal' HIJ relationship (fig. 1a).

Case II. R.E. A 29-year-old male complaining of precordial twinges of pain: BP 202/104. Bcg: diminished amplitude with early 'H' and accentuated J_R with J segmentation. Following five days of tranquilizer (Valium®) therapy while continuing usual ambulatory activity: BP 138/86. Bcg: HIJ relationship is restored to 'normal' (fig. 1b).

Case III. C.C. A 46-year-old male with history of convulsive seizures two days prior to examination: BP 164/120. Bcg: impaired amplitude and configuration in the control

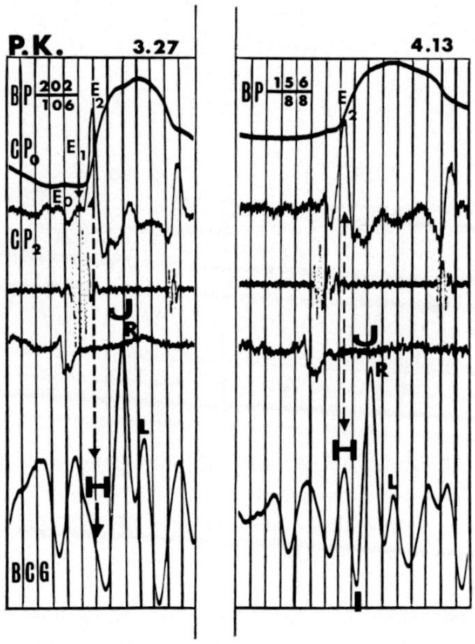

Fig. 2. P.K. Age 66. Female. 3.27.72; BP 202/106. 'H' is seen as a slur on the descending limb of the isometric wave followed by a markedly accentuated J_R. 4.13.72 (following diuretic and tranquilization therapy): BP 156/88. H is clearly evolved and in more normal relation to the peak (E_2) of the ejection wave in the second derivative of the carotid pulse (CP_2). HI remains relatively diminished – hence, is followed by an accentuated J_R.

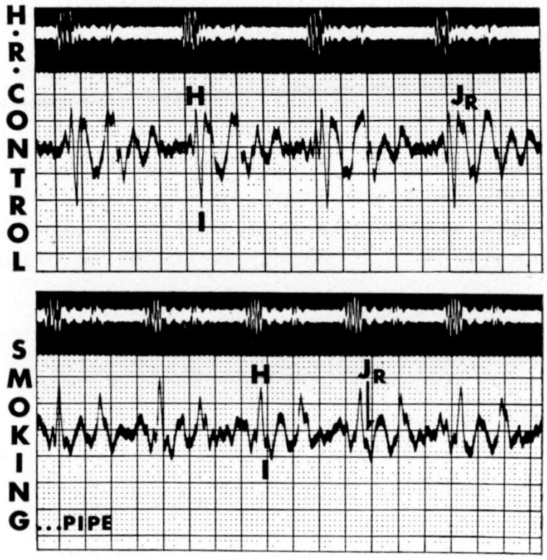

Fig. 3. H. R. Age 40. Male. An inveterate pipe smoker complaining of precordial pains. One pipe-full of tobacco caused overall deterioration in amplitude and configuration of all segments of HIJ – ostensibly a reflection of increased peripheral vascular resistance.

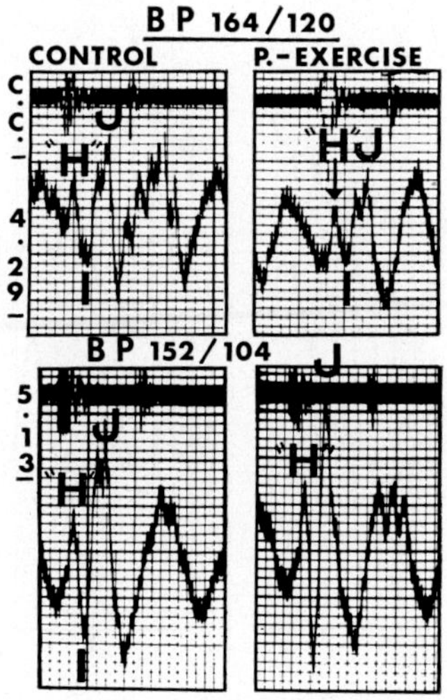

Fig. 4. C. C. (same as fig. 1 c): Note the further depression of the overall pattern following exercise during the hypertensive phase as contrasted with its accentuation following tension reduction.

study were restored by combined vasodilatation [pentaerythritol tetranitrate (PETN)] and antipressor (Rauwiloid®) drug therapy (fig. 1c).

Case IV. P.K. A 66-year-old female complaining of fatigue and palpitations and exhibiting hypernatremia: BP 202/106. Bcg: early 'H'-accentuated J_R. Following tranquilizer (Valium®) and diuretic (Hygroton®) therapy: BP 156/88. Bcg: evolution of the true H from the trough of the earlier 'H' I is evident (fig. 2).

Case V. H.R. A 40-year-old male complaining of precordial pains ostensibly related to excessive pipe smoking with resulting increased peripheral vascular resistance [26, 27]. The overall deterioration of the Bcg following one pipe-full of tobacco is readily evident (fig. 3).

Comments

Several points deserve emphasis. The first and most cogent is the dynamic sensitivity of the myocardium to the hypertensive afterload particularly ap-

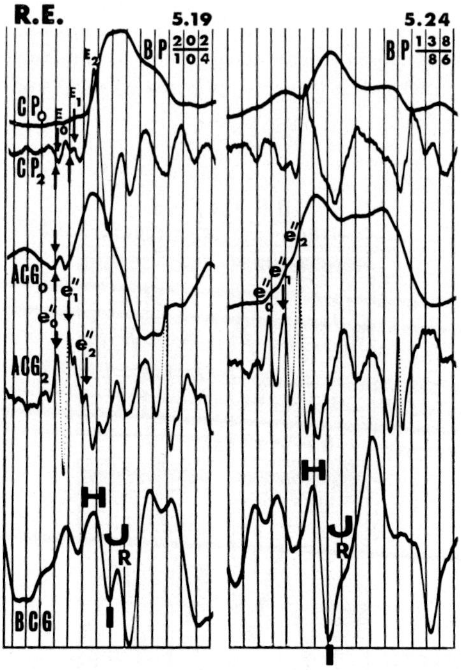

Fig. 5. R.E. (same as in fig. 1b): This suggests correlation of the alterations in the Bcg with those in the second derivative of the ACG involving dominantly the third component of the ejection wave (e''_2) – deteriorated in the hypertensive phase and prominent in the normotensive phase.

parent in cases I and II – significant for their young age with its minimum of morphologic alteration and prompt response to the most benign of therapeutic measures. Also, despite lack of difference in the PEP/LVET ratio [23] between the two phases, its stress implication is suggested by its further Bcg deterioration following exercise (fig. 4) instead of its usual enhancement [22]. The second point is the apparently corresponding alteration of the second derivative of the ejection (E) wave in the ACG revealed in case II (fig. 5) where the third, usually dominant, e''_2 segment shows deterioration in the hypertensive phase suggesting the same shift of the basic dynamics of ejection as previously described in coronary artery disease [24]. The third point is the possible Bcg reflection of alteration in catecholamine content within the myocardium suggested following Rauwolfia therapy [25].

Summary

It has been proposed that hypertension does affect the form of the Bcg pattern as recorded with the HF (a) DB Bcg consistent with known physiologic principle. This is illustrated with patients serving as their own control. The dominant alterations are those of diminished amplitude and shift in pattern form from a 'normal' HIJ relation in the normotensive phase to one of early 'H'-accentuated J_R in the hypertensive phase. Exercise tends to enhance the normality of the former and produce further deterioration in the latter. Correlated deterioration of initial dynamics in the ACG is suggested.

Acknowledgements

I wish to express my gratitude to Miss FAITH CARSO for her dedicated assistance in the performance of these studies and to Mr. WILLIAM RONIN for his artistic preparation of the illustrations.

References

1 ARBEIT, S. F. and LINDNER, N.: A new full frequency range calibrated ballistocardiograph. Amer. Heart J. *48:* 52–59 (1959).
2 BRAUNWALD, E.; ROSS, J., jr.; GAULT, J. H.; MASON, D. T.; MILLS, C.; GABE, I., and EPSTEIN, S. E.: Assessment of cardiac function. Ann. intern. Med. *70:* 369–399 (1969).
3 DOCK, W. and TAUBMAN, F.: Some technics for recording the ballistocardiogram directly from the body. Amer. J. Med. *7:* 751–755 (1949).
4 EICHNA, L. W.: Hypertension and the heart. Bull. N.Y. Acad. Med. (second series) *45:* 809–818 (1969).

5 Gleason, W.L. and Braunwald, E.: Studies on the first derivative of ventricular pressure pulse in man. J.clin.Invest. *41:* 80–91 (1962).

6 Harrison, W.K.; Friesinger, G.C.; Johnson, S.L.; Ross, R.S., and Johns, R.J.: Relation of the ballistocardiogram to left ventricular pressure measurements in man. Amer.J.Cardiol. *23:* 673–678 (1969).

7 Mason, D.T.; Sonnenblick, E.H.; Covell, J.W.; Ross, J., jr., and Braunwald, E.: Assessment of myocardial contractility in man. Relationship between the rate of rise and developed pressure throughout left ventricular contraction. Circulation *36:* suppl.II, pp.183–184 (1967).

8 Ross, J., jr. and Braunwald, E.: Study of left ventricular function in man by increasing resistance to ventricular ejection with angiotensin. Circulation *31:* 739–749 (1964).

9 Ross, J., jr.; Covell, J.W.; Sonnenblick, E.H., and Braunwald, E.: Contractile state of the heart characterized by force-velocity relations in variably afterloaded and isovolumic beats. Circulat.Res. *18:* 149–163 (1966).

10 Sarnoff, S.J.; Braunwald, E.; Welch, G.H., jr.; Case, R.B.; Stainsby, W.N., and Macruz, R.: Hemodynamic determinants of oxygen consumption of the heart with special reference to the tension time index. Amer.J.Physiol. *192:* 148–156 (1958).

11 Scarborough, W.R. and Talbot, S.A.: Proposals for ballistocardiographic nomenclature and conventions. Revised and extended. Report of Committee on Ballistocardiographic Terminology. Circulation *14:* 435–450 (1956).

12 Shillingford, J.G.: Hemodynamic effects of acute myocardial infarction in man. Progr.cardiovasc.Dis. *9:* 571–593 (1967).

13 Shillingford, J.G. and Thomas, M.: Cardiovascular and pulmonary changes in patients with myocardial infarction in an intensive care and research unit. Amer.J. Cardiol. *20:* 484–493 (1967).

14 Sonnenblick, E.H. and Downing, S.E.: Afterload as a primary determinant of ventricular performance. Amer.J.Physiol. *204:* 604–610 (1963).

15 Spann, J.F., jr.; Buccino, R.A.; Sonnenblick, E.H., and Braunwald, E.: Contractile state of cardiac muscle obtained from cats with experimentally produced ventricular hypertrophy and heart failure. Circulat.Res. *21:* 341–354 (1967).

16 Starr, I.: Does the presence of hypertension itself increase force BCG abnormality? Proc. 14th annu. Meet.Ballistocard.Res.Soc., Atlantic City 1970; Bibl.cardiol., vol.27, pp.36–39 (Karger, Basel 1971).

17 Starr, I. and Noordergraaf, A.: Ballistocardiography in cardiovascular research. Physical aspects of the circulation in health and disease (North Holland Publishing, Amsterdam; Lipincott, Philadelphia 1967).

18 Urschell, C.W.; Covell, J.W.; Sonnenblick, E.H.; Ross, J., jr., and Braunwald, E.: Myocardial mechanics in aortic and valvular regurgitation: the concept of instantaneous impedance as a determinant of the intact heart. J.clin.Invest. *47:* 867–883 (1968).

19 Wallace, A.G.; Skinner, N.S., jr., and Mitchell, J.H.: Hemodynamic determinants of the maximal rate of rise of left ventricular pressure. Amer.J.Physiol. *205:* 30–48 (1963).

20 Weissler, A.M.; Harris, W.S., and Schoenfeld, C.D.: Bedside technics for the evaluation of ventricular function in man. Amer.J.Cardiol. *23:* 577–583 (1969).

21 WINER, N. J.: The second derivative of the carotid pulse as an aid in high-frequency (acceleration) direct body BCG segment notation; in Ballistocardiography and cardiovascular performance. Proc. 11th annu. Meet. Ballistocard. Res. Soc., Atlantic City 1966. Bibl. cardiol., vol. 19, pp. 103–109 (Karger, Basel 1967).

22 WINER, N. J.: High-frequency (acceleration) direct body ballistocardiography: a new concept in its application and diagnosis of early acute myocardial infarction: in Proc. 2nd World Congr. Ballistocard. cardiovasc. Dynamics, Oporto 1969. Bibl. cardiol., vol. 26, pp. 52–65 (Karger, Basel 1970).

23 WINER, N. J.: High-frequency (acceleration) direct body ballistocardiography. The rule of H-J_R reciprocity; in Proc. 8th Europ. Congr. Ballistocard., Ljubljana 1971. Bibl. cardiol. (Karger, Basel, in press).

24 WINER, N. J.: Some preliminary observations on the correlation of the high-frequency (acceleration) direct body ballistocardiogram with the apexcardiogram, carotid pulse and their derivatives; in Proc. 15th annu. Meet. Ballistocard. Res. Soc., Atlantic City 1971. Bibl. cardiol., vol. 29, pp. 74–85 (Karger, Basel 1972).

25 WINER, N. J.: Unpublished observation.

26 WINER, N. J.: The BCG reflections of the pathophysiology of the heart beat as recorded with the high-frequency (acceleration) direct body BCG; in Proc. 6th Europ. Congr. Ballistocard., London 1967. Bibl. cardiol., vol. 21, pp. 102–115 (Karger, Basel 1968).

27 WOOD, J. E.: Effect of smoking on the peripheral circulation in relation to environmental temperature. Ann. N.Y. Acad. Sci. *90:* 114–118 (1960).

Author's address: NAHUM J. WINER, M.D., 103 East 78th Street, *New York, NY 10021* (USA)

Proc. 16th ann. Meet. Ballistocard. Res. Soc., Atlantic City 1972;
Bibl. Cardiol. *32:* 58–71 (Karger, Basel 1973)

Physiologic Expressions of Cardiac Dynamics by High-Frequency (Acceleration) direct Body Ballistocardiography[1]

N. J. WINER

Lenox Hill Hospital, New York City, N.Y.

The purpose of this presentation is to indicate that the high-frequency (acceleration) direct body ballistocardiogram (HF [a] DB Bcg) does reflect cardiac dynamics in terms of physiologic principle affirmed by other recognized methods. It is presented in the context of three basic groups: (A) electrical or conductivity effects; (B) effects of preload (Frank-Starling mechanism) and afterload; (C) contractility.

Method

The physical characteristics of the HF (a) DB Bcg [2, 6], the nature of its record and application [28, 29] have been previously described and will not be repeated in the interests of space. Recordings were made with the Sanborn Twin-Beam standardized by a beam displacement of 1 cm by 1 mV for overall dynamic perspective and serial comparison and an Electronics for Medicine DR 8, correlating different parameters for accurate segment notation and qualitative characterization.

Studies

A. Electrical or Conductivity Effects

1. Pathway of excitation. A beat of supraventricular (atrial or nodal) origin which follows a normal path of excitation is dynamically different from one

[1] This study was aided by a grant from the Florence G. Heller Foundation and, in part, by the Xerox Corporation, BERTRAM HOFFBERGER, and the family of Mr. SAMUEL W. HUROWITZ in his memory.

of ventricular origin whose pathway, unless arising from the area of the Bundle of His, is abnormal. The former, even if premature (PAC) will, at most, present a pattern of diminished amplitude but be, qualitatively, of normal configuration if the ventricular myocardium itself is not ischemic. The latter, certainly if premature (PVC), is not only diminished in amplitude but shifts its configuration to one of early 'H' and deeply segmented J (J_R-J_L) representing full myocardial dynamic depression (fig. 1). It has been variously characterized as one of disorderly fractionate excitation with diminished dynamics [27]; decreased acceleration and peak outflow rate of blood comparable to that of paradoxic pulsation [21]; asynergy depending on site, origin and timing [7] whose depression is reflected by adverse hemodynamic measurements [12]. This may be otherwise illustrated here (fig. 2) by a previously described case of intermittent left bundle branch block [30] whose depressed performance [12] is physiologically reflected in its decreased dp/dt [25] and increased preejection period/left ventricular ejection time ratio (PEP/LVET) [26].

2. Bowditch ('Treppe') phenomenon. The enhanced level of contractility and sympathetic stimulation [9] with increased dp/dt [25] recently related to intracellular sodium and calcium [14] is manifest following the sudden con-

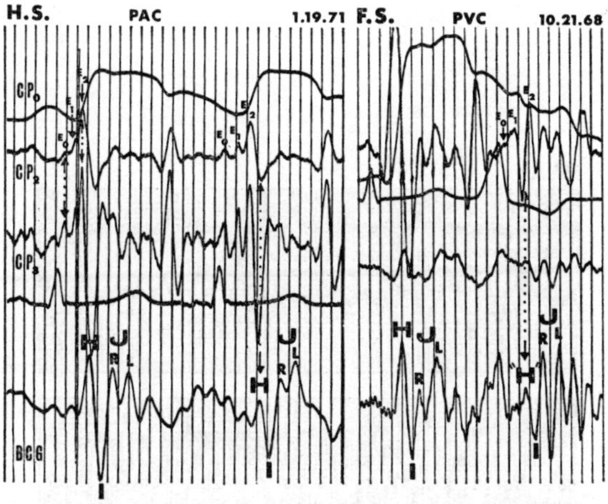

Fig. 1. H.S. Premature atrial beat with normal pathway of excitation is characterized by a normal configuration though of diminished amplitude and is in normal relation to the peak of the ejection wave (E_2) in the second derivative of the carotid pulse (CP_2). This is in contrast to the PVC in F.S. which represents full myocardial depression characterized by overall diminished amplitude with early 'H' relative to E_2 in CP_2 and is followed by a deeply segmented J. In both cases, the hearts are ostensibly normal.

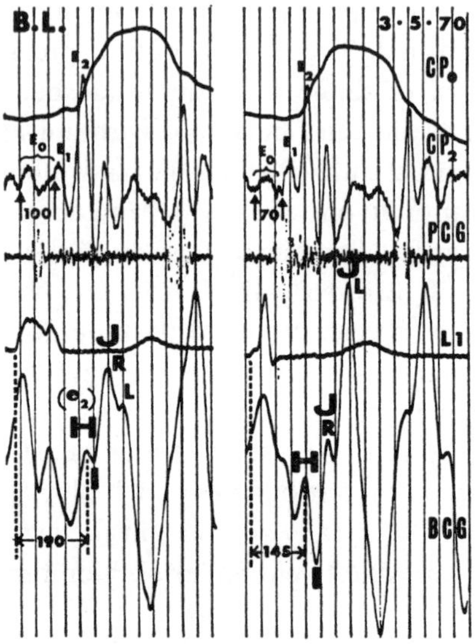

Fig. 2. B.L. (arteriosclerotic heart disease): alteration of forces in intermittent left bundle branch block. Note transitional improvement as well as overall amplitude followed by shift of J peak from J_R to J_L. This is correlated with reduction of 45 msec in the q_{Ecg}-H interval as well as the first of the two fundamental phases of the isovolumetric period (E_o) in CP_2 of 30 msec.

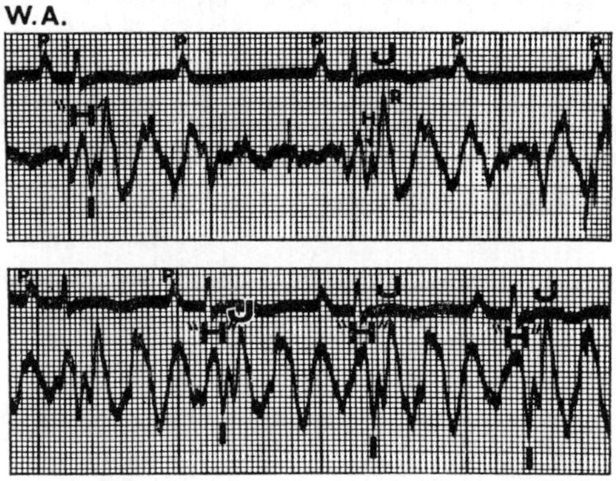

Fig. 3. W.A. (Ebstein's anomaly): Bowditch ('Treppe') phenomenon. Note progressive enhancement of the Bcg patterns of about one third more following transition from 2:1 block to normal response despite shortened diastolic filling periods.

version from second degree block to normal conduction despite shorter diastolic filling periods (fig. 3).

3. Post-extrasystolic potentiation. Studies attributing its augmentation to increased contractility [13, 32], its inverse relation to prematurity and time to maximal potentiation [5] without essential increase in cardiac output is visualized here in the 'piggy-back' effect of two extrasystoles where the second produces still further augmentation by occurring before the potentiation of the first has subsided (fig. 4).

4. Potentiation by interval ratio. The inverse relationship of dynamics to the RR_1/RR_2 ratio of the preceding two beats in atrial fibrillation is similarly illustrated (fig. 5) [22].

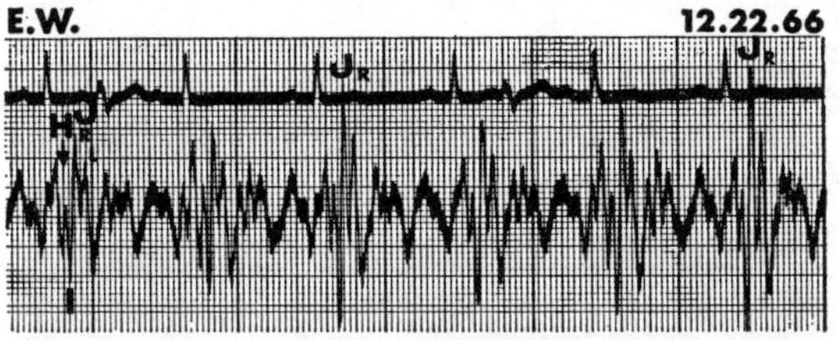

Fig. 4. E.W. (arteriosclerotic heart disease): post-extrasystolic potentiation. Note progressive enhancement of the second beat following the first interpolated extrasystole with superimposition of a second interpolated extrasystole before the effects of the first had subsided resulting in still further potentiation of the pattern.

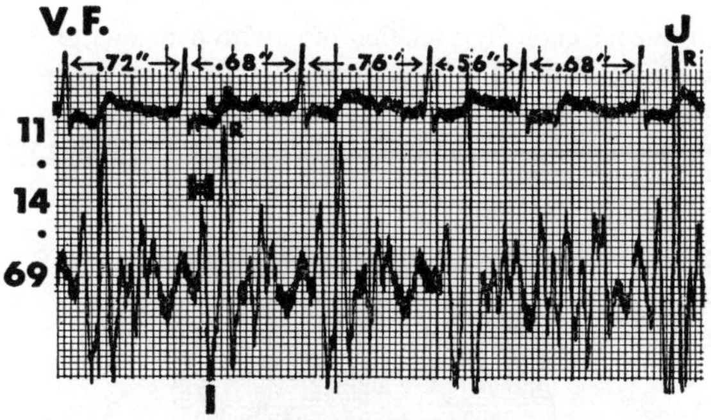

Fig. 5. V.F. (combined aortic and mitral valvular disease with atrial fibrillation): dynamics are inversely related to the RR_1/RR_2 ratio preceding it. Note two R-R intervals of the same 0.68 sec. The first is preceded by one of 0.72 sec; the second by 0.56 sec. The J_R segment following the latter is strikingly potentiated over that of the first. Note, also, that the amplitude of each beat is inversely related to the period of diastolic filling preceding it.

B. Preload (Frank-Starling) Mechanism

1. While the increased force of contraction by increasing diastolic filling has been described in the compensatory pause [5], it may be better demonstrated in the varying diastolic filling periods of atrial fibrillation (fig. 5).

2. Atrial 'kick'. The booster function of the atrium raising the end-diastolic volume and pressure, thereby maintaining cardiac output even at rest [18] is evident in complete block where the 'H' I wave as well as overall amplitude are augmented as the atrial impulse approaches that of the ventricle (fig. 6).

3. Pulsus alternans. The relation of alternating strength of contraction to alternating end diastolic fibre length [19] concordant with left ventricular end diastolic volume as determined by biplane ventriculography [10] as well as equating alternating pressure, stroke volume and flow velocity by Doppler flowmeter [3] negates WIGGERS' early concept of alternate deletion of contractile units [27]. Here, the more normal HIJ relationship of the stronger

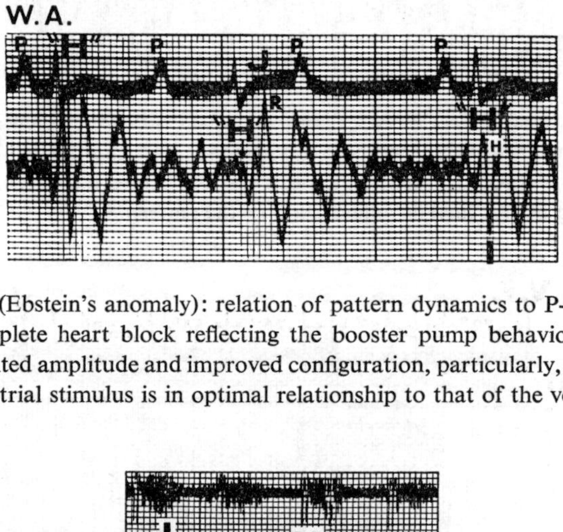

Fig. 6. W.A. (Ebstein's anomaly): relation of pattern dynamics to P-R interval in the presence of complete heart block reflecting the booster pump behavior of the atrium. Note the augmented amplitude and improved configuration, particularly, of the initial 'H'I wave when the atrial stimulus is in optimal relationship to that of the ventricle.

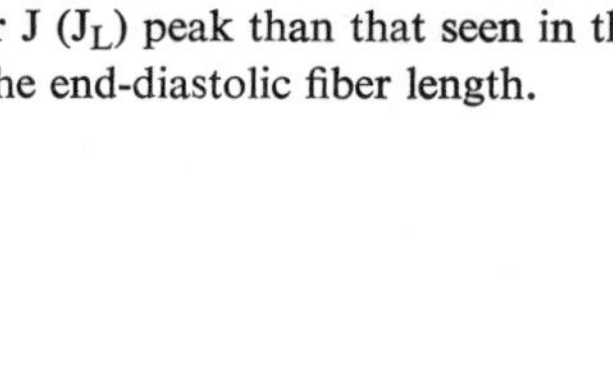

Fig. 7. E.L. (aortic stenosis): pulsus alternans. Note the steeper ascending and descending slopes of the initial HI segment of the stronger beat with J_R seen as a slur on the ascending limb to a later J (J_L) peak than that seen in the weaker beat. This is attributed to the alternation in the end-diastolic fiber length.

beat with its greater amplitude, steeper HI slope and J_R slur on the ascending limb to J_L with greater intensity of the heart sound is evident (fig. 7).

4. Mitral stenosis. Where severe, impaired ventricular diastolic filling is reflected by the essential absence of the initial HI segment (fig. 8). Following valvulectomy, this is promptly restored. Of notable interest is the Bcg sensitivity to the physiological nuances of increasing heart rate with its increasing left atrial gradient and mitral valve flow rate [1, 17] resulting in a transient increase in the initial HI segment despite, even prolonged, electrocardiographic reflections of ischemia. Similarly, the diminished availability of blood to the ventricle by decreased venous return due to peripheral vasodilatation – whether following nitroglycerin or sympathetic nervous system weakness – and reflected by overall diminished amplitude and possibly J segmentation has been previously described [16, 31].

5. *Afterload.* The clinical problems related to this are those of hypertension, valvular and subvalvular aortic stenosis. The first of these is broadly reviewed elsewhere in this volume and will not be repeated here. The effect of valvular aortic stenosis is illustrated in two ways: first, the progressive loss of the initial HI segment accompanied by antecedent accentuation of the 'A' wave

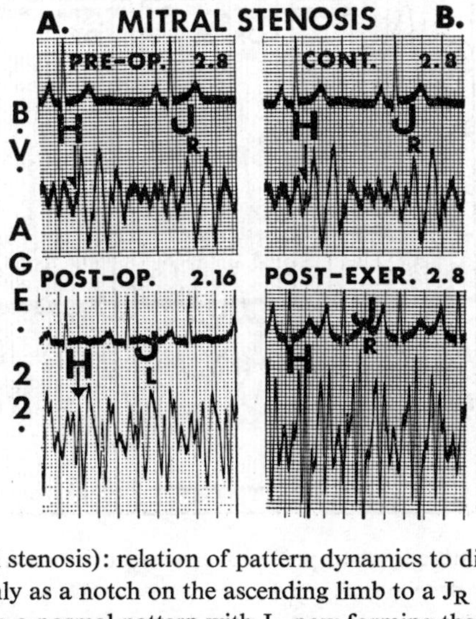

Fig. 8. B.V. (mitral stenosis): relation of pattern dynamics to diastolic filling. *A* 2.8.72, pre-op.: H appears only as a notch on the ascending limb to a J_R peak. 2.16.72, post-op.: HIJ is fully restored to a normal pattern with J_L now forming the peak of J reflecting the prompt response to the increased ventricular filling as well as the good underlying contractile state of the myocardium. *B* Increasing atrial gradient with exercise: control, same as A; Post exercise: There is marked accentuation of HI though J_R still forms the peak of J.

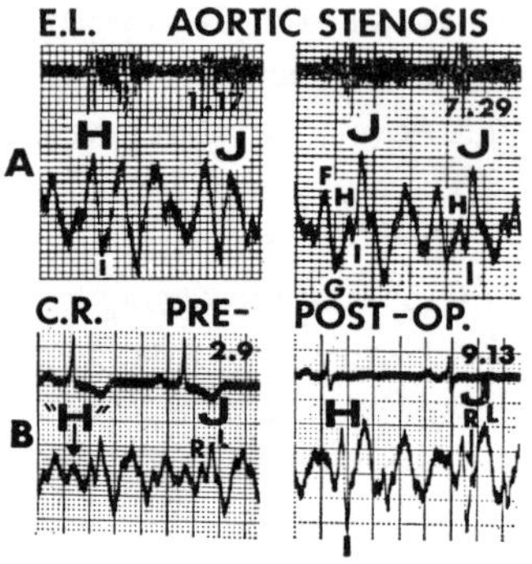

Fig. 9 A–B. A. E.L. (aortic stenosis): 1.17: prominent HIJ during pulsus alternans phase same as that in figure 7; 7.29 (6 weeks prior to exitus): marked diminution in HI with accentuation of antecedent 'A' wave (F-G) with S_4. *B* C.R. (aortic stenosis): 2.9.66. Preop.: complaints of frequent angina on exertion. Note overall diminution in amplitude with early 'H' and segmented J; 9.13.66. 6 months post-op.: The HIJ pattern is markedly improved in amplitude and presents a normal configuration. The slow progressive restoration post-operatively emphasizes the slow dynamic responses to reduction in afterload as against that to an increase in preload (mitral stenosis).

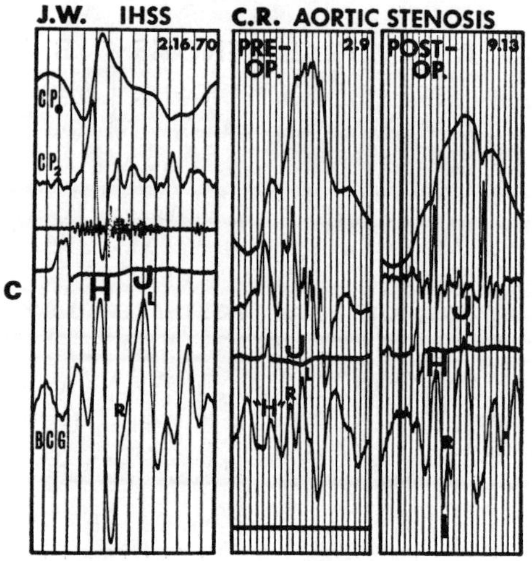

Fig. 9 C. J.W. (idiopathic hypertrophic subaortic stenosis) versus C.R. (aortic stenosis, same as 9B): In IHSS, despite tachycardia and ischemic ST-T depression in the accompanying Ecg, the Bcg pattern is augmented and of normal configuration. This is correlated with a rapid rise in the carotid pulse wave (CP_0, CP_2). In contrast, C.R. presents an abnormal Bcg pattern correlated with a slow rise in the carotid pulse containing the 'shudder' of stenosis.

(fig. 9 A); second, its gradual recovery following valvulectomy (fig. 9 B). In contrast to these, the early rapid pressure rise in idiopathic hypertrophic subaortic stenosis [4] is well reflected in the Bcg as it is in the carotid pulse (fig. 9 C).

C. Contractility

Here, the DB (a) Bcg offers its greatest potential in reflecting the intrinsic state of the myocardium whether altered by ischemia, necrosis or drugs and may serve as a yardstick of further depression or recovery. Physiologically,

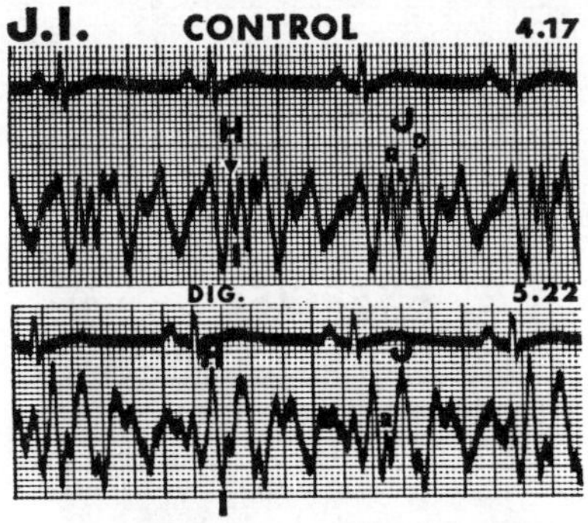

Fig. 10. J.I. (paroxysmal atrial fibrillation of no known etiology): control: the initial HI wave is diminished and is followed by deep J segmentation of which J_R is the more prominent segment; post-digitalization: HI is markedly improved with a normal HIJ segment interrelationship reflecting improved myocardial contractility.

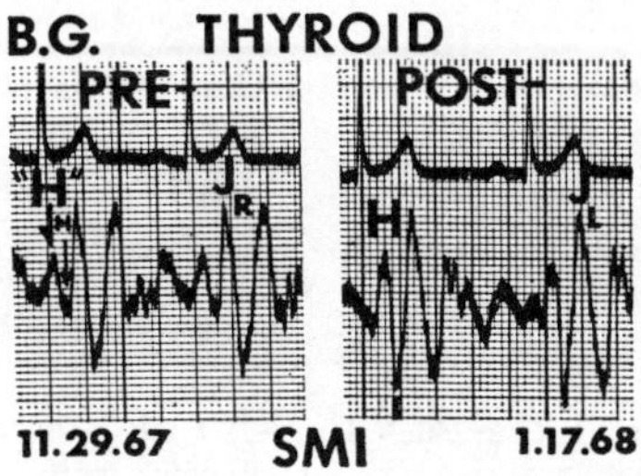

Fig. 11. B. G. (neurocirculatory astenia with depressed basal metabolism; BMR): 11.29.67: the Bcg pattern is characterized by an early 'H' followed by accentuation of J_R with a note that the true H is seen as a slur submerged in the trough of 'H'I J_R; 1.17.6. (following thyroid administration): the pattern is restored to normal with a corrected q_{Ecg}-H interval of 0.16 sec as against 0.08 sec before therapy.

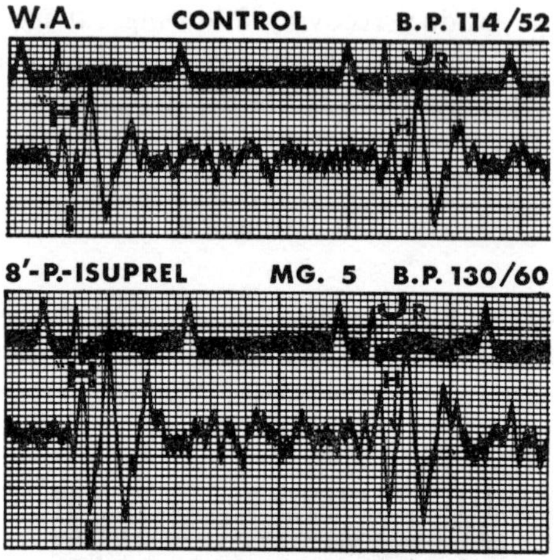

Fig. 12. W.A. (Ebstein's anomaly in 2:1 block): administration of isoproterenol (mg. $\overline{V}$ sublingual) produced marked improvement of all segments of the Bcg pattern within 8 min of administration.

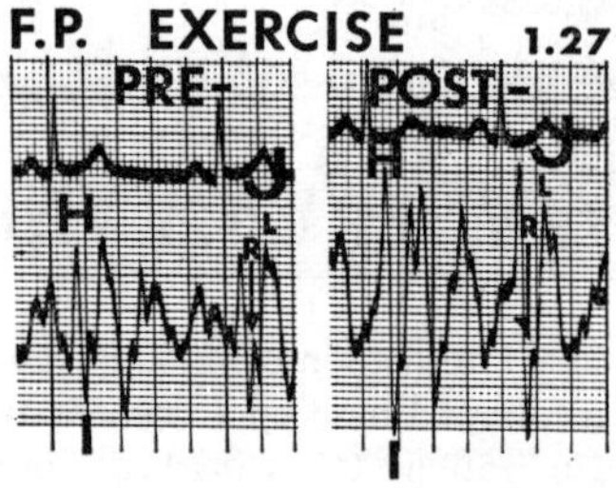

Fig. 13. F.P. (normal heart): effect of exercise on Bcg dynamics. The normality of the Bcg pattern – amplitude and configuration – is further accentuated following a double Master two-step test reflecting the amplifying effect of the release of catecholamines.

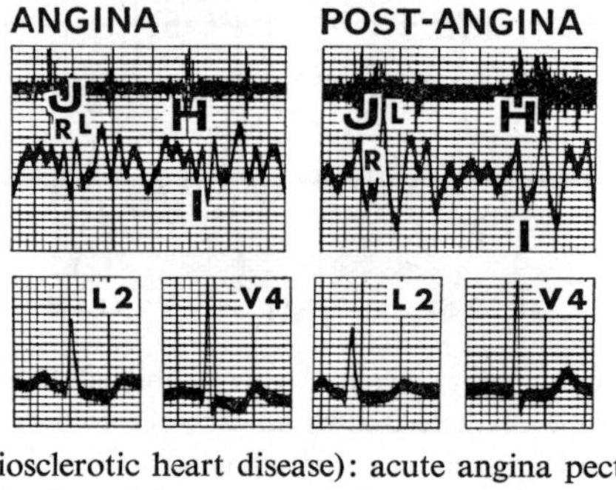

Fig. 14. M.L. (arteriosclerotic heart disease): acute angina pectoris. Note the overall diminution in Bcg amplitude and deep segmentation of J correlated with ST-T depression in the Ecg. These are restored within minutes of the cessation of pain.

the ventricular function curves relating left ventricular end-diastolic pressure and stroke volume have been noted to be shifted upward and to the left [24] as has the shift in force-velocity relation with increase in V_{max} and P_o [23]. The resulting increased contractility implying increased dp/dt and reduced time to peak dp/dt has been emphasized [15]. These are reflected in the Bcg by such inotropes as digitalis (fig. 10), thyroid (fig. 11), isoproterenol (fig. 12) and the catecholamines released by exercise (fig. 13). Conversely, the myocardial depression in angina [27] with its paradoxic pulsation [8, 11] and its

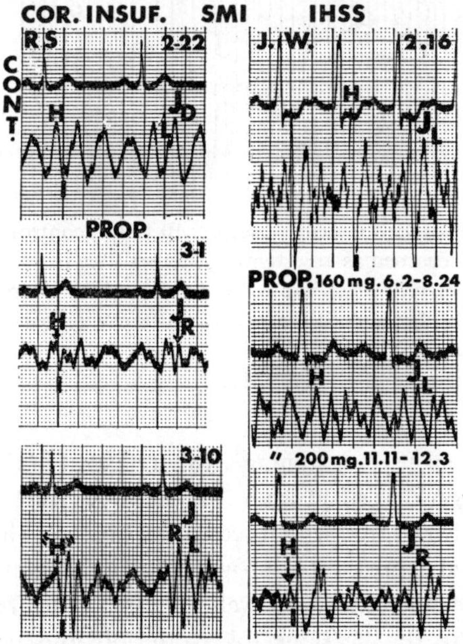

Fig. 15. R.S. Age 40, male (arteriosclerotic heart disease; three vessel disease established by coronary arteriography). Effect of propranolol on myocardial dynamics during therapy for angina: 2.22: control: while the Bcg pattern was not wholly normal for reasons of diminished negative phase, HI is of relatively good amplitude and bears a normal time relationship to the peak of the ejection wave (E_2) in CP_2 and to q_{Ecg} of 0.16 sec; 3.1 (1 h following administration of propranolol totalling 70 mg): note overall diminution in amplitude with H still in normal time relationship to q_{Ecg}; 3.6 (following continued administration of propranolol of 40 mg/day): the appearance of early 'H' with shortening of the interval from q_{Ecg} is regarded as representative of full myocardial depression. J.W. Effect of propranolol in the therapy of IHSS (same as fig. 9): accompanying progressive slowing in heart rate, there is diminution in the amplitude of the Bcg, particularly, of the initial HI wave with H slightly earlier relative to the peak of the ejection wave (E_2) in CP_2 and shortening of the q_{Ecg}-H interval from 0.16 to 0.12 sec while the J peak similarly shifts from that of J_L to J_R.

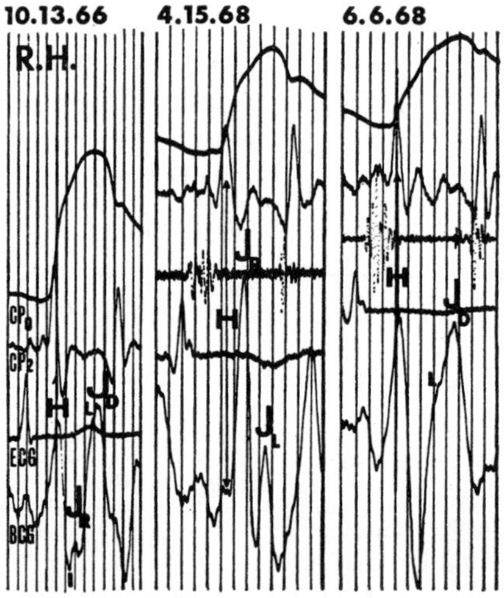

Fig. 16. R.H. (arteriosclerotic heart disease): 10.13.66: control: two years post myocardial infarction and regarded as an essentially normal Bcg pattern; 4.15.68: acute myocardial infarction: H is fully deteriorated and followed by deep J segmentation with marked accentuation of J_R; 6.6.68: the overall pattern with particular attention to the initial HI wave is restored.

asynergic implications [8] is instantaneously reflected in the Bcg by the same pattern of depression described above in the PVC (early 'H' – deeply segmented J) and is fully restored with its cessation (fig. 14). This can be simulated by such a myocardial depressant as propranolol in the treatment of idiopathic hypertrophic subaortic stenosis as well as angina and reserved by its discontinuance (fig. 15). By the same token, the obvious depression by myocardial necrosis results in the same pattern through the transitional alterations involving both H and J waves which, unless residual scarring is definitive, may be restored gradually through convalescence to its initial normal state (fig. 16).

Summary

The thesis is proposed that the HF (a) DB Bcg can reflect the physiology of myocardial dynamics. This has been illustrated in the dynamic impairment of aberrant conduction or prematurity of contraction, on the one hand, or its augmentation by increasing frequency of contraction or post-extrasystolic potentiation, on the other. It has been shown to reflect the advantages of the Frank-Starling mechanism and the impairment of increasing afterload. Its sensitivity to the inotropism of certain drugs and exercise and, conversely, the myocardial depression of angina, necrosis or certain myocardial depressants as propranolol has been indicated. All of these attest to the basic validity of its application to clinical cardiac evaluation.

Acknowledgments

I wish to express my gratitude to Miss FAITH CARSO for her dedicated assistance in the performance of these studies and to Mr. WILLIAM RONIN for his artistic preparation of the illustrations.

References

1 ARANI, D.T. and CARLETON, R.D.: The deleterious role of tachycardia in mitral stenosis. Circulation *36:* 511–516 (1967).

2 ARBEIT, S.F. and LINDNER, N.: A new full frequency range calibrated ballistocardiograph. Amer. Heart J. *45:* 52–59 (1959).

3 BENCHIMOL, A.; SCHUMACHER, J., and DESSER, K.B.: Concordant right and left heart pressure and flow velocity alternans. Chest *61:* 183–184 (1972).

4 BRAUNWALD, E.; LAMBREW, C.T.; ROCKOFF, S.D.; ROSS, J., jr., and MORROW, A.G.: Idiopathic Hypertrophic Subaortic Stenosis: description of the disease based upon an analysis of 64 patients. Circulation *29:* suppl. IV, p. IV–I (1964).

5 CHEVALIER-CHOLAT, A.M.; TORRESENI, J.; SAADJIAN, A.; HEUILLET, G., and JOUVE, A.: Post extra systolic potentiation during coupled stimulation of the heart. J. Electrocard. *4:* 341–346 (1971).

6 DOCK, W. and TAUBMAN, F.: Some technics for recording the ballistocardiogram directly from the body. Amer. J. Med. *7:* 751–755 (1949).

7 EBER, L.M.; COOKE, J.M., and GORLIN, R.: The dynamic characterization of ventricular premature beats in man. J. clin. Invest. *47:* 26A (1968).

8 EDDLEMAN, E.E., jr. and LANGLEY, J.O.: Paradoxical pulsations of the precordium in myocardial infarction and angina pectoris. Amer. Heart J. *63:* 579–581 (1962).

9 GLEASON, W.L. and BRAUNWALD, E.: Studies of the first derivative of the ventricular pressure pulse in man. J. clin. Invest. *41:* 80–91 (1962).

10 GLEASON, W.L. and BRAUNWALD, E.: Studies of Starling's law of the heart. VI. Relationship between left ventricular end diastolic volume and stroke volume in man with observations on the mechanism of pulsus alternans. Circulation *25:* 841–848 (1962).

11 HARRISON, T.R. and HUGHES, L.: Precordial systolic bulges during anginal attacks. Trans. Ass. Amer. Phys. *71:* 174–185 (1958).

12 HERMAN, M.V. and GORLIN, R.: Implications of left ventricular asynergy. Amer. J. Cardiol. *23:* 538–547 (1969).

13 HOFFMAN, B.F.; BINDLER, E., and SUCKLING, E.: Post extrasystolic potentiation of contraction in cardiac muscle. Amer. J. Physiol. *185:* 95–102 (1956).

14 LANGER, G.A.: The intrinsic control of myocardial contraction. Ionic factors. New Engl. J. Med. *285:* 1065–1071 (1971).

15 MASON, D.T.: Usefulness and limitations of the rate of rise of intraventricular pressure (dp/dt) in the evaluation of myocardial contractility in man. Amer. J. Cardiol. *23:* 516–527 (1969).

16 MASON, D.T. and BRAUNWALD, E.: The effect of nitroglycerin and amylnitrite on arteriolar and venous tone in the human forearm. Circulation *32:* 755–766 (1965).

17 MITCHELL, J.H.; GILMORE, J.P., and SARNOFF, S.J.: The transport function of the atrium. Factors influencing the relation between mean left atrial pressure and left ventricular end diastolic pressure. Amer. J. Cardiol. *9:* 237–247 (1963).

18 MITCHELL, J.H. and SHAPIRO, W.: Atrial function and the hemodynamic consequences of atrial fibrillation in man. Amer. J. Cardiol. *23:* 556–567 (1969).

19 MITCHELL, J.H.; SONNENBLICK, E.H., and SARNOFF, S.J.: Pulsus alternans. Alternating end diastolic fiber length as a causative factor. Fed. Proc. *20:* 129 (1961).

20 ROSS, J., jr.: The assessment of myocardial performance in man by hemodynamic and cineangiographic technic. Amer. J. Cardiol. *23:* 511–515 (1969).

21 RUSHMER, R.F.: Initial ventricular impulse. A potential key to cardiac evaluation. Circulation *29:* 268–283 (1964).

22 SHABETAI, R.; UTHER, J.B.; PETERSON, K.L., and ROSS, J., jr.: Potentiation of contraction by premature activation in patients with normal and abnormal left ventricular function. Amer. J. Cardiol., Abstract. 21st annu. sci. Sess. Amer. Coll. Cardiol., p. 291 (1972).

23 SONNENBLICK, E.H.: The mechanics of myocardial contraction; in CONN and BRILLER The myocardial cell, pp. 173–250 (University of Pennsylvania Press, Philadelphia 1966).

24 STARLING, E.H.: The Linacre Lecture on the Law of the Heart, given at Cambridge, 1915 (Longmans, London 1918).

25 WALLACE, A.G.; SKINNER, N.S., jr., and MITCHELL, J.H.: Hemodynamic determination of the maximal rate of rise of left ventricular pressure. Amer. J. Physiol. *205:* 30–36 (1963).

26 WEISSLER, A.M.; HARRIS, W.S., and SCHOENFELD, C.D.: Bedside technics for the evaluation of ventricular function in man. Amer. J. Cardiol. *23:* 577–583 (1969).

27 WIGGERS, C.G.: Dynamics of ventricular contraction under abnormal conditions. Circulation *5:* 321–348 (1952).

28 WINER, N.J.: High-frequency (acceleration) direct body ballistocardiography: a new concept in its application and diagnosis of early acute myocardial infarction. Proc. 2nd World Congr. Ballistocard. cardiovasc. Dynamics, Oporto 1969. Bibl. cardiol., vol. 26, pp. 52–65 (Karger, Basel 1970).

29 WINER, N.J.: The second derivative of the carotid pulse as an aid in high-frequency (acceleration) direct body BCG segment notation. Proc. 11th annu. Meet. Ballistocard. Res. Soc., Atlantic City 1966. Bibl. cardiol., vol. 19, pp. 103–109 (Karger, Basel 1967).

30 WINER, N.J.: The effect of bundle branch block on cardiac dynamics as recorded with the high-frequency (acceleration) direct body ballistocardiograph. Proc. 14th annu. Meet. Ballistocard. Res. Soc., Atlantic City 1970. Bibl. cardiol., vol. 27, pp. 25–35 (Karger, Basel 1971).

31 Winer, N.J.: The BCG reflections of the pathophysiology of the heart beat as recorded with the high-frequency (acceleration) direct body BCG. Proc. 6th europ. Congr. Ballistocard., London 1967. Bibl. cardiol., vol. 21, pp. 102–115 (Karger, Basel 1968).
32 Woodworth, R.S.: Maximal contraction, 'staircase' contraction, refractory period and compensatory pulse of the heart. Amer. J. Physiol. *8:* 213–249 (1902).

Author's address: Nahum J. Winer, M.D., 103 East 78th Street, *New York, NY 10021* (USA)

Proc. 16th ann. Meet. Ballistocard. Res. Soc., Atlantic City 1972;
Bibl. Cardiol. *32:* 72–82 (Karger, Basel 1973)

Determination of Cardiac State[1]

S. Fich, B. Min, W. Welkowitz, D. Jaron and A. Kantrowitz

Department of Electrical Engineering, Rutgers University
Department of Surgery, Sinai Hospital, Detroit, Mich.

Introduction

This paper presents a method for determining cardiac state from *in vivo* measurements of pressure and flow under two conditions of after-loading. The left ventricle is modelled as a pressure source having an internal impedance. It is shown that the parameters of the pressure source are related to the heart muscle parameters. Stress-length variations under conditions of drug induced nerve blockage and simulated heart failure are calculated. Evaluation of the muscle parameters may have practical value in assessing cardiac state.

Analysis

Using results based upon muscle mechanics as given in the appendix, separate expressions for time and frequency domain representations of left ventricular pressure, for both the isometric and isotonic states of muscle contraction, are obtained for the thin semi-ellipsoidal model assumed for the left ventricle shown in figure 1. In this figure, σ_1 and σ_2 are the longitudinal and transverse circumferential stresses, and a and b are the semi-major and semi-minor axes of the ellipse. The stress-length variation of the heart muscle can be expressed by a single equation in the frequency domain by using a piecewise Fourier analysis with time limits corresponding to the durations of the isometric and isotonic states [7]. The result yields a frequency domain representation of the heart as a pressure source, P_g, with an internal imped-

[1] This research was supported in part by a grant from the Rutgers Research Council and USPHS grant HE-11173.

ance, Z_g. These are shown in figure 2 where the valve impedance is denoted by Z_v, the left ventricular pressure by P_{lv}, and the pressure, flow, and input impedance at the root of the aorta by P_a, Q_a, and Z_a. All the above quantities are phasors. Although Z_v is a nonlinear impedance, the phasor representation is shown to be valid when all the components have the same fundamental frequency [7].

The phasor equation that characterizes the performance of the left ventricle is

$$P_{lv} = P_g - Z_g Q_a \cdot \tag{1}$$

The maximum isovolumic stress, $\bar{\sigma}$, and the dynamic variation in length, $\bar{l}$, in the direction of the semi-minor axis, for the assumed uniform semi-ellipsoidal section, are related to the source parameters by the following equations:

$$\bar{\sigma} = \frac{K_1 P_g}{\sqrt{Z_g}}, \tag{2}$$

$$\bar{l} = \frac{K_2}{\sqrt{Z_g}}, \tag{3}$$

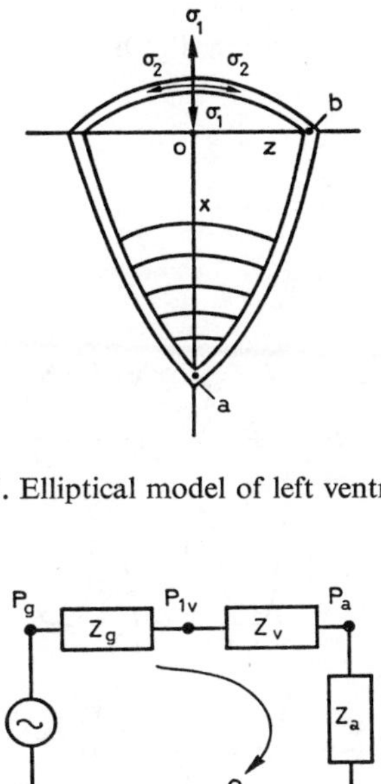

Fig. 1. Elliptical model of left ventricle.

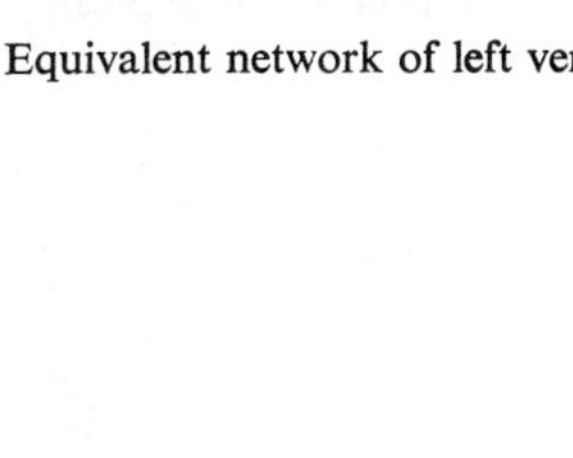

Fig. 2. Equivalent network of left ventricle.

where K_1 and K_2 are constants depending upon the dimensions of the section, and P_g and Z_g are the magnitudes of the Fourier components at the fundamental frequency. Since the dynamic variations in length in the direction of the semi-major axis are negligible compared with those along the semi-minor axis in the assumed configuration, it follows that l is proportional to the square root of the dynamic change in volume.

It can be seen from equations 2 and 3 that if P_g and Z_g can be calculated in the *in vivo* state, the relation between the maximum isovolumic stress and the dynamic length variation can be obtained. This is accomplished by varying the effective load on the heart using an intra-aortic balloon pump to change the aortic impedance. Time domain records of left ventricular pressure and flow are recorded for the unassisted condition and also during the initial or second cycle of pumping. This procedure eliminates the effects of the physiological controls upon the muscle parameters because the time constants of the cardiovascular control paths have been estimated to be much greater than the period required for one cycle pumping in a dog with a heart rate of about 150 beats/min [8]. The effect of pumping on aortic pressure, left ventricular pressure, and aortic flow is shown in figure 3.

Using prime and double prime symbols to denote the phasor components of left ventricular pressure and aortic flow before and after pumping, the components of P_g and Z_g, as calculated from equation 1 are as follows:

$$P_g = \frac{P'_{lv} Q''_a - P''_{lv} Q'_a}{Q''_a - Q'_a}, \tag{4}$$

$$Z_g = \frac{P_g - P'_{lv}}{Q'_a} = \frac{P_g - P''_{lv}}{Q''_a} \tag{5}$$

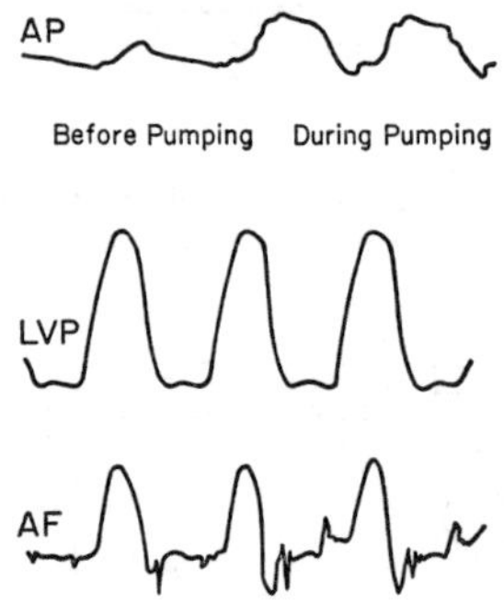

Fig. 3. Effects of intra-aortic pump on aortic pressure, left ventricular pressure, and aortic flow.

where P_g and Z_g are assumed constant during one cycle of pumping because of the relation between the period and the control system time constants. P_{lv} and Q_a, with appropriate primed notation, are the Fourier series components calculated from the time domain records of left ventricular pressure and aortic flow.

Experimental Procedure

Mongrel dogs weighing between 25 and 32 kg were anesthetized with sodium pentobarbitol (25 mg/kg), and intubated for artificial respiration. The balloon was introduced through the femoral artery into the descending aorta. Either the electrocardiogram or the left ventricular pressure was used to synchronize the operation of an external driving system with the cardiac cycle. Left ventricular and aortic pressures were measured by polyethylene catheters placed in the left ventricle through the apex, and in the root of the aorta through the carotid artery. The balloon was introduced through the femoral artery into the descending thoracic artery.

In addition to using the balloon pump for determining the pressure and impedance phasors of the equivalent pressure source, the pump was also used to relieve left ventricular failure that was induced by ligating all branches of the anterior descending coronary artery. The heart was considered to be in failure when cardiac output decreased by at least 40%, systolic blood pressure, by 30% or more of the preligation values, and when left ventricular end-diastolic pressure increased to 12 mm Hg or more. These are the same criteria as used by JARON *et al.* [6] in simulating cardiac failure. Timing is important, and perhaps critical, in the therapeutic use of the pump.

Results

If an attempt is made to determine P_g and Z_g from the measurements indicated in equations 4 and 5, it is found that P_g and Z_g vary with time. The reason for this is that P_g and Z_g are the Fourier components of essentially time-varying functions. As previously noted, Fourier analysis is valid in this case because all the variables have the same fundamental frequency. Variations of P_g and Z_g with time can be substantially reduced by the use of drugs to block the sympathetic and parasympathetic nerve control systems. For this purpose, Inderal (0.5 mg/kg) and atropine (3 mg/kg) were intravenously injected, for 3 and 5 min, respectively. The effectiveness of blockage was checked by noting that injection of epinephrine produced much smaller changes in both the heart rate and left ventricular pressure than the corresponding changes produced by the same injection in the normal state. Figure 4 shows the fluctuations of P_g and Z_g with time before and after nerve blockage. The fluctuations from the mean value are reduced by about 75% for P_g and 60% for Z_g for a period of 1 h after injection.

Figures 5 and 6 show the Fourier components of P_g and Z_g for the first five harmonics for both the control and failure states. Experiments on several dogs showed considerable fluctuations in the ratio of the failure to the control values for a given harmonic. It should be noted that equation 3 does not apply for the constant term in the Fourier series. Hence, it is possible to have an increase in volume for the failing heart with an increased value of the

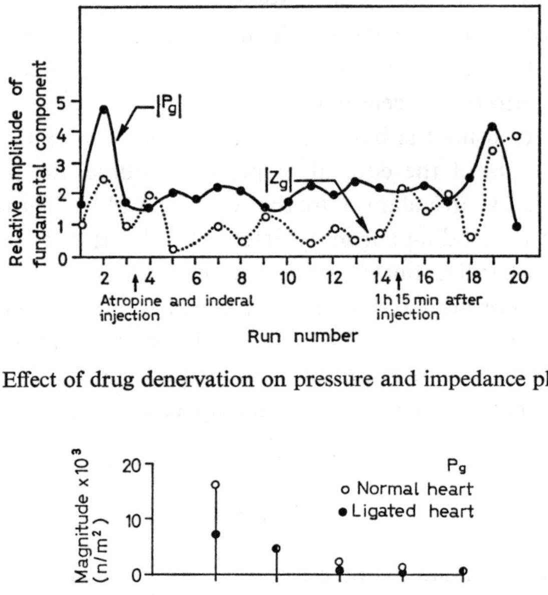

Fig. 4. Effect of drug denervation on pressure and impedance phasors.

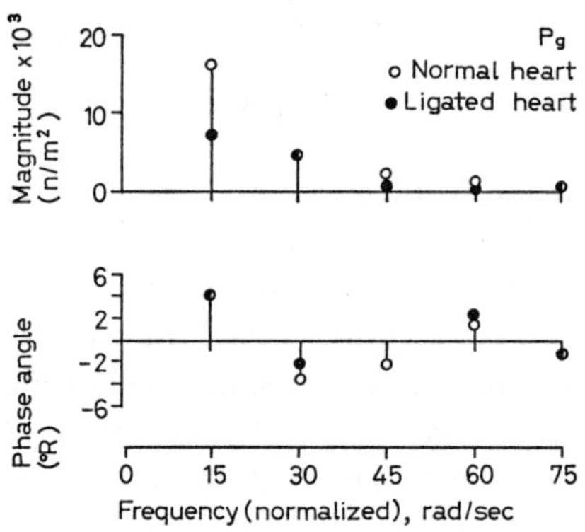

Fig. 5. Fourier components of source pressure.

fundamental component of Z_g. Figure 7 shows the source pressure, $P_g(t)$ constructed from its Fourier components.

Figure 8 shows the calculated stress-length variations for four dogs for the normal and nerve blocked conditions. Curves A and D are for the nerve-blocked state, and curves B and C are for the normal condition. These results are in reasonable agreement with those given by COTTEN and BAY [3]. Figure 9 shows the effect of epinephrine injection (0.9 μ/kg) on the stress-length function. The injection of epinephrine increased the calculated maximum isovolumic stress above that for the control state for each value of dynamic length. This result is also in reasonable agreement with the experiments of SARNOFF [10]. All calculations were based on equations 2 and 3.

Figure 10 shows a linear variation in measured fundamental component

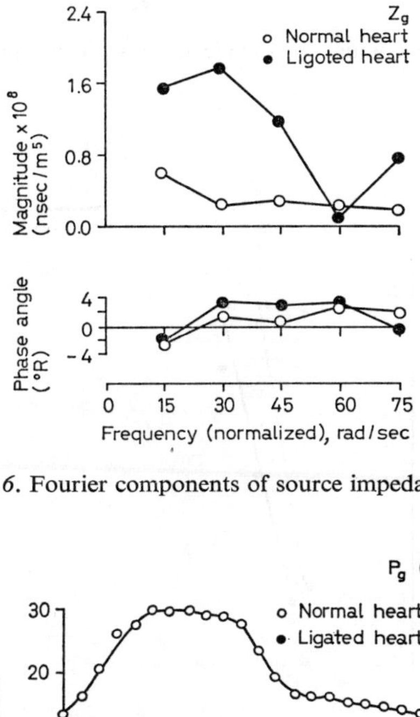

Fig. 6. Fourier components of source impedance.

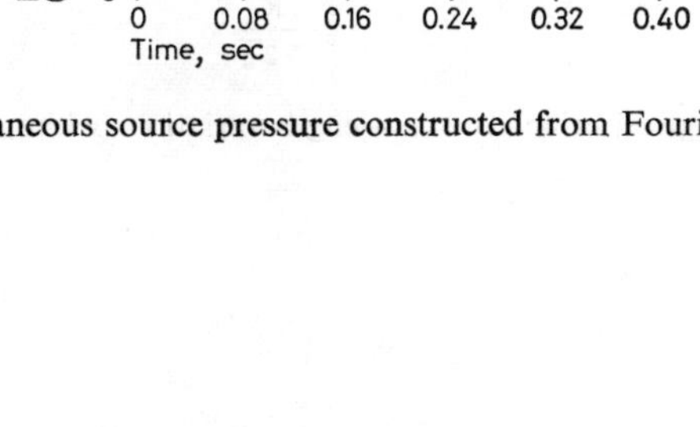

Fig. 7. Instantaneous source pressure constructed from Fourier components.

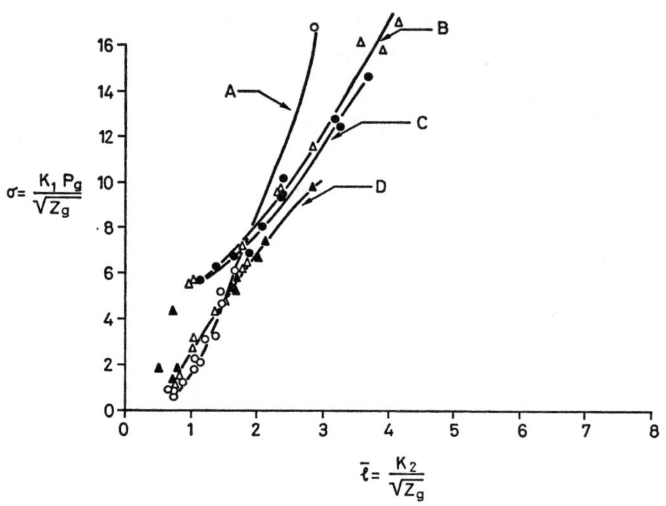

Fig. 8. Variation of maximum isovolumic stress with dynamic change in length for 4 dogs.

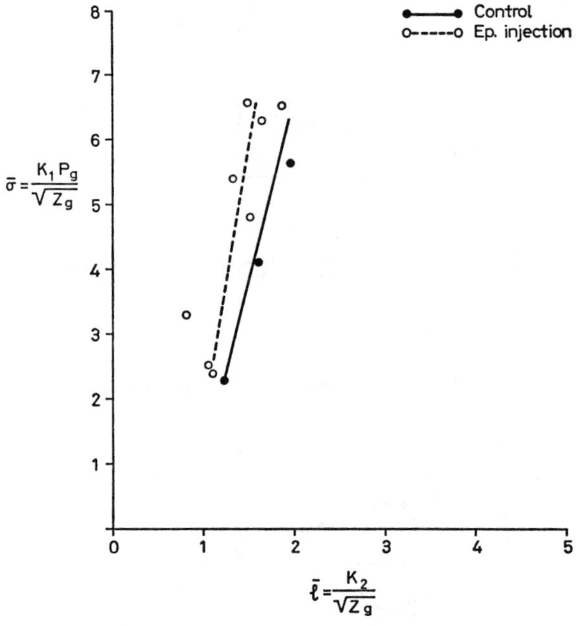

Fig. 9. Effect of epinephrine on stress-length variation (without denervation).

of aortic flow (proportional to stroke volume for the case of constant heart rate in the nerve blocked condition) with $\frac{1}{Zg}$ Left ventricular volume variation, proportional to $\frac{1}{Zg}$, can be shown to be directly proportional to the left ventricular end-diastolic pressure [2]. It has also been shown that a linear relationship exists between end-diastolic pressure and end-diastolic volume [1]. Hence, a linear relation exists between $\frac{1}{Zg}$ and end-diastolic pressure. It follows that figure 10 implies a linear relation between stroke

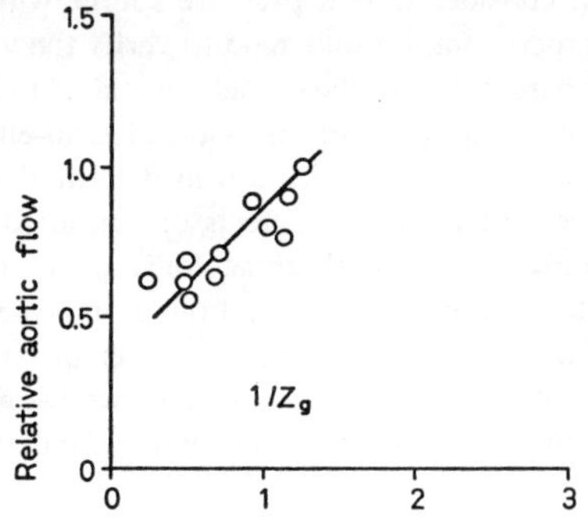

Fig. 10. Aortic flow as a function of end diastolic pressure.

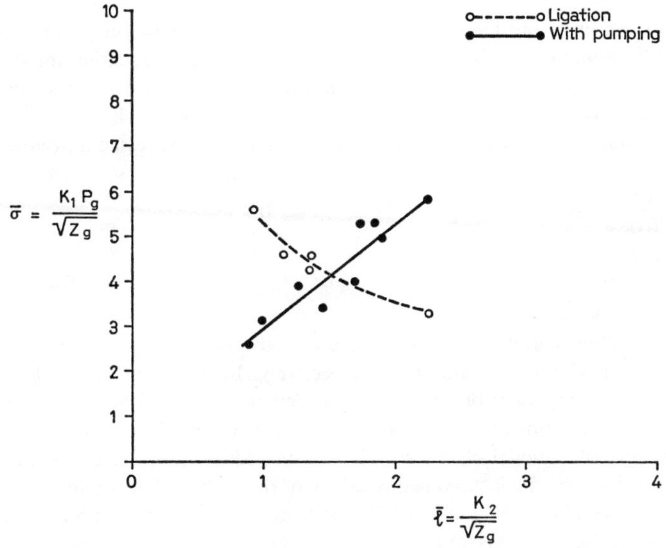

Fig. 11. Stress-length variation for ligated coronary arteries before and after balloon pumping.

volume and end-diastolic pressure. This result is given by GUYTON [4]. Figure 11 shows the calculated stress-length variations for induced failure before and after therapeutic pumping. In the case of therapeutic pumping, an attempt is made to optimize cardiac assistance [6].

Summary

A model of the heart, considered as a pressure source with an internal impedance, has been presented, and experimental results tend to verify the validity of this model. The analysis indicates that the parameters of the model are related to the maximum isovolumic stress and the dynamic length variation of an assumed semi-elliptical section of the left ventricle. Hence, the model may find application in determining stress-length variations from *in vivo* hemodynamic measurements. Effects of various drugs upon the calculated stress and length are consistent with pharmacologic data. The effect of intra-aortic assistance upon the calculated stress-length variations is indicated. Data from two experiments suggest that the Starling mechanism persists after pharmacologic denervation. If further experiments substantiate the initial results, an effective method for assessing both the cardiac state and the effect of cardiac assistance may be made available.

Appendix

The following in an outline of the derivations of equations 1–3 in the text.

Using Hill's equation for the isometric phase and Carlson's equation for the isotonic phase of ventricular muscle contraction, and applying Laplace's equation to the assumed ellipsoidal model of the left ventricle having a very thin wall as shown in figure 1, the instantaneous ventricular pressure during contraction can be expressed as follows [5, 7, 9]:

$$p_1(t) = \frac{A(t)}{l(t)} \frac{b}{a} \alpha\bar{\sigma}\, t \qquad 0 < t < t_e, \qquad \text{(A-1)}$$

$$p_2(t) = \frac{A(t)}{l(t)} \sigma(t) - \frac{1}{2} \frac{A(t)}{v(t)} rq(t) \qquad t_e < t < T, \qquad \text{(A-2)}$$

where the subscripts 1 and 2 refer respectively to the isometric and isotonic phases of contraction having duration t_e and $T-t_e$, respectively. In equations A-1 and A-2, $\sigma(t)$ is the instantaneous component of pulsatile circumferential stress, $\bar{\sigma}$ is its maximum value, α is the elastic constant of the series elastic element in the model of the muscle, a and b are constants in Hill's model of the muscle, r is the constant in Carlson's model of the muscle, h(t) and l(t) are the instantaneous values of the wall thickness and the semi-minor axis of the assumed ellipsoidal model of the left ventricle, and A(t) is approximately equal to 1.45 h(t) as derived by SHASTRI [11].

The periodic time-varying functions can be expressed by a Fourier series with complex coefficients as follows:

$$p_{lv}(t) = p_1(t) + p_2(t) = \sum_{-\infty}^{\infty} P_{lv}(n\,\omega_1)\,\varepsilon^{jn\omega_1 t}, \qquad \text{(A-3)}$$

$$A(t) = \sum_{-\infty}^{\infty} A(n\omega_1)\,\varepsilon^{jn\omega_1 t}, \qquad \text{(A-4)}$$

$$l(t) = \sum_{-\infty}^{\infty} l(n\omega_1)\,\varepsilon^{jn\omega_1 t}, \qquad \text{(A-5)}$$

$$v(t) = \sum_{-\infty}^{\infty} V(n\omega_1)\,\varepsilon^{jn\omega_1 t}, \qquad \text{(A-6)}$$

$$\sigma(t) = \sum_{-\infty}^{\infty} \overline{\sigma}(n\omega_1)\,\varepsilon^{jn\omega_1 t}, \qquad \text{(A-7)}$$

where $pl_v(t)$ is the instantaneous left ventricular pressure, $v(t)$ is the stroke volume, and ω_1 is the fundamental repetition rate common to all of the above functions.

The following derivation is valid for the case where all the time-varying functions have the same fundamental repetition rate which in this case is the heart rate [7]. Considering only the fundamental Fourier components ($n = 1$), and eliminating subscripts, the phasor component of left ventricular pressure is given by

$$P_{lv} = \frac{A}{l}\,\overline{\sigma}\left[\frac{1}{T}\int_0^{t_e} \frac{b}{a}\,\alpha t\,\varepsilon^{-j\omega_1 t}\,dt + \frac{1}{T}\int_{t_e}^{T} dt\right] - \left[\frac{1}{2}\frac{A}{V}\,r\right]\frac{1}{T}\int_{t_e}^{T} q(t)\,\varepsilon^{-j\omega_1 t}\,dt. \qquad \text{(A-8)}$$

Since $q(t) = 0$ when $0 < t < t_e$,

$$\frac{1}{T}\int_{t_e}^{T} q(t)\,\varepsilon^{-j\omega_1 t}\,dt = \frac{1}{T}\int_0^{T} q(t)\,\varepsilon^{j\omega_1 t}\,dt = Q_a, \qquad \text{(A-9)}$$

where Q_a is the flow phasor.

Equation A-8 can be written as

$$P_{lv} = \frac{A}{l}\,\overline{\sigma}\left[\frac{1}{T}\int_0^{t_e} \frac{b}{a}\,\alpha t\,\varepsilon^{-j\omega_1 t}\,dt + \frac{T - t_e}{T}\right] - \frac{1}{2}\frac{A}{V}\,r\,Q_a. \qquad \text{(A-10)}$$

Equation A-10 has the form

$$\hat{P}_{lv} = \hat{P}_g - \hat{Z}_g\,\hat{Q}_a, \qquad \text{(A-11)}$$

where all the terms are phasors as in equation 1 of the text.

Since only variations in the length along the semi-minor axis are considered, the stroke volume is proportional to the square of the change in length. Hence,

$$\bar{l} = \frac{K_2}{\sqrt{Z_g}}. \tag{A-12}$$

Substitution of equation A-12 into equation A-10 yields

$$\bar{\sigma} = \frac{K_1 P_g}{\sqrt{Z_g}}, \tag{A-13}$$

where all terms represent absolute values.

References

1 BENEKEN, J.E.W.: A mathematical approach to cardiovascular function. Report No. 2-4-5/6 (Institute of Medical Physics, Utrecht 1965).

2 DAVSON, H. and EGGLE, M.G.: Starling's human physiology, vol. 14, p. 163 (Lea & Febiger, Philadelphia 1968).

3 COTTEN, M.D. and BAY, F.: Direct measurements of changes in cardiac contractile force. Amer. J. Physiol. *187:* 122 (1956).

4 GUYTON, A.C.: Textbook of medical physiology; 2nd ed., p. 334 (Saunders, Philadelphia 1964).

5 HILL, A.V.: The heat of shortening and dynamic constants of muscles. Proc. roy. Soc. B *126:* 136 (1938).

6 JARON, D. *et al.:* Measurements of ventricular load phase angle as an operating criterion for in series assist devices. Trans. Amer. Soc. Artif. Int. Organs, vol. 16, pp. 466–471 (1970).

7 MIN, B.: Analysis and optimization of balloon pumping; Ph.D. thesis, Department of Electrical Engineering, Rutgers University, New Brunswick, N.Y. (1972).

8 PURI, N.N. and GIDO, J.F.: Control systems for circulating assist devices, pp. 3–4 (University City Science Center, Philadelphia 1968).

9 RITCHIE, J.M. and WILKIE, D.R.: Dynamics of muscular contraction. J. Physiol., Lond. *143:* 104 (1958).

10 SARNOFF, S.J.: Myocardial contractility as described by ventricular function curves: observations on Starling's law of the heart. Physiol. Rev. *35:* 108 (1955).

11 SHASTRI, J.S.: A Thevenin equivalent model of the left ventricle derived from hemodynamic measurements obtained by use of a ventricular assist pump; Ph.D. thesis, Department of Electrical Engineering, Rutgers University (1969).

Authors' addresses: S. FICH, B. MIN and W. WELKOWITZ, Department of Electrical Engineering, Rutgers University, *New Brunswick, NJ 08903;* D. JARON and A. KANTROWITZ, Department of Surgery, Sinai Hospital of Detroit, *Detroit, MI 48235* (USA)

Proc. 16th ann. Meet. Ballistocard. Res. Soc., Atlantic City 1972;
Bibl. Cardiol. *32:* 83–93 (Karger, Basel 1973)

The HI Slope of the Ballistocardiogram Used to Compute Indices of Myocardial Contractility in Man[1]

J. BAAN

Cardiovascular-Pulmonary Division, Department of Medicine,
Hospital of the University of Pennsylvania, Philadelphia, Pa

Introduction

Indices of myocardial contractility are most commonly derived from the phasic isovolumic left ventricular pressure P_V. Except for maximum derivative, dP_V/dt, most of these indices involve the computed velocity (V_{CE}) of the so called contractile element of the sarcomere based on the assumption of a 2 or 3 element muscle model [11]. These computations and models have been recently criticized on fundamental grounds by several workers [8, 13]. In addition, the limitations of the indices were delineated by some of the proponents [11]. As a corollary to the latter study, maximal dP_V/dt was found to be the most sensitive of the pressure-derived indices [PARMLEY, personal commun.] and also one of the most effective indices of ventricular performance [12], even though it was more dependent on preload than some of the others [11].

Other indices of the contractile state of the left ventricle have been found to derive from the phasic aortic root blood flow ($\dot{Q}$) during the early phase of ejection [7, 14]. Partly because this quantity is difficult to measure and partly because of the apparent success of the pressure-derived indices mentioned above, this work did not attract much attention. Nevertheless, it has been shown in dogs that some of the flow-derived indices, in particular maximal acceleration ($d\dot{Q}/dt$), are equally or more sensitive to variations in contractility than maximal dP_V/dt [7, 9]. We have confirmed this work and found also that the same is true for maximal aortic dp/dt [BAAN *et al.*, 2a]. However, the dependence of the flow-derived indices on preload and afterload has not

[1] Supported by National Institutes of Health grant HE-08805.

been clearly established yet [9]. Phasic blood flow at the aortic root is directly related to the actual velocity of shortening of left ventricular muscle fibers, the maximal value of which was recently found to be a very good index of contractility in man [10]. This actual shortening velocity is the subject of recent fundamental studies on isolated muscle fibers [3]. Even though these studies appear to be promising, we feel that the most important advantage of contractile indices derived from flow over those derived from isovolumic ventricular pressure lies in the fact that flow involves mass motion, which may be transmitted to the body in such a way that it can be measured non-invasively. The ballistocardiogram (Bcg) seemed to be the obvious of such noninvasive methods and the results in patients are reported in this study.

Theoretical Considerations

A mathematical relationship between the HI slope of the Bcg and acceleration of flow $d\dot{Q}/dt$ during the first 25 msec of ejection was derived previously [1] and resulted in the following approximate formula (the notation $d\dot{Q}/dt$ replaces the originally used d^2Q/dt^2):

$$M \frac{d^3Y}{dt^3} = - 3/2\, \varrho\, c \frac{d\dot{Q}}{dt} \cos \alpha, \tag{1}$$

where M is the body mass, d^3Y/dt^3 the slope of the acceleration Bcg, ϱ the blood density, c the apparent pulse wave velocity in the ascending aorta, and α the angle between ascending aortic axis and head-foot axis. In the model used, the expansion of the elastic aortic wall was assumed to be parallel [1]. If this assumption is replaced by the perhaps more realistic one of a tapering expansion (i.e., maximal expansion at the aortic valve, linearly decreasing with distance to the wave front), then the velocity at which the center of gravity of the expansion travels equals 1/3 c. This contrasts with the original value of 1/2 c for the velocity of the center of gravity of the parallel expansion and would modify equation 1 to the same relation without the factor 3/2. Interestingly, this would likewise modify the relation originally derived from equation 1 for the aortic pressure derivative dp/dt:

$$M \frac{d^3Y}{dt^3} = - \frac{3}{2} S \frac{dp}{dt} \cos \alpha, \tag{2}$$

where S is the aortic cross-sectional area. Without the factor 3/2 and integrated once, this relationship states that the force (Md^2Y/dt^2) as recorded by the Bcg is numerically equal to the head-foot component of the force

(S p cos α) generated by the pressure in the aortic root! Nevertheless, our experimental observations fitted the original equations much better and thus we kept the factor 3/2 in the formulas. This problem will be discussed below.

Methods

Studies were performed in patients who underwent right and left heart catheterization by conventional techniques [1] for evaluation of cardiac disease. We succeeded in obtaining simultaneous records of aortic root blood velocity and Bcg in five patients; of aortic root pressure and Bcg in twelve. Phasic velocity tracings were obtained from a No. 8 Carolina Medical Electronics catheter-tip velocity probe except in one patient where an SE Laboratories Mills-type probe was used. All catheters were introduced through the right brachial artery and advanced to the ascending aorta. The linearity of the Carolina Medical probe was tested *in vitro* over a range from 0 to 25 cm/sec and found to be better than 2%. Frequency response of the flow meter (CME501D) was flat within 5% from 0 to 10 Hz. The velocity signal was converted into a calibrated flow signal in each patient by means of the cardiac output, obtained by dye dilution method with indocyanine green and a Gilford densitometer. In view of the noise of the records, flow acceleration was obtained by hand-drawn slopes.

The apparent pulse wave velocity (c) in the ascending aorta was assumed to be 4 m/sec in all patients [6].

Aortic root pressures (p) were obtained through 125-cm-long No. 7 or 8 Sones catheters using Statham P23Db transducers. The frequency response of these catheter-manometer systems was determined using a sine wave pressure generator and found to be flat within 5% from 0 to 30 Hz. However, because these catheters were always used for selective coronary angiography up to 45 min prior to Bcg recording, the possibility existed that remnants of the radiopaque dye introduced damping of the signal, causing the catheters to resonate at lower frequencies (from 15 Hz upward). To a certain extent, these frequencies are also generated by catheter whip. To minimize the error from resonance artefacts, dp/dt was determined graphically. In one patient the pressure tracing was damped so much that his case was excluded from the study. In the flow studies, pressures were also recorded through the saline-filled lumen of the velocity probe but since this lumen is very narrow, the pressure tracings were always damped too much to be useable.

Cross-sectional area (S) of the ascending aorta was calculated from the diameter as measured from the ventriculogram. Forty to 50 ml of 63% Renovist was power injected into the left ventricle via a No. 7 or 8 Lehman catheter. Cineangiograms were obtained with a 6–9 dual field General Electric image intensifier. The image of the catheter (enlarged about 10 times) was used to obtain the enlargement factor. The angle α between aortic axis and head-foot axis was also estimated from the angiograms.

Bcg was obtained from a ballistobed especially constructed to fit the fluoroscopy table, which is equipped with a Cordis body rotating device (Rotacor). This bed has been described previously [1]. The acceleration Bcg ($\ddot{Y}$) was recorded with a Kistler accelerometer (305 A) with a frequency response flat to at least 30 Hz. Recordings were obtained during apnea, usually at the mid-expiratory level. The value of d^3Y/dt^3 was obtained graphically from the slope of the HI segment. If the I wave was double or the HI slope was not constant, the maximum value was taken.

All signals were inscribed on an Electronics for Medicine photographic recorder (DR-8) at high paper speed (100 mm/sec).

Results

Preliminary results of simultaneous Bcg and flow or pressure were reported previously in three patients: one with flow and two with pressure [1]. Sample records of the other 13 patients are shown in figures 1, 2 and 4.

Thus, in the previous study [1] we showed Bcg and blood velocity obtained with the SE Laboratories velocity probe in a patient with coronary artery disease. It also demonstrated the simultaneity of the HI slope with the onset of ejection. In this patient, beat-to-beat variations in HI slope (d^3Y/dt^3) and flow acceleration ($d\dot{Q}/dt$) fitted the mathematical relationship (equation 1) to a satisfactory degree, especially during the recovery from a Valsalva maneuver.

The flow studies in the other four patients were obtained with the Carolina Medical Electronics (CME) velocity probe and a sample is shown in a patient with mitral insufficiency in figure 1. In general, although the Bcg was irregular and not normal in most cases, the HI slope was easily identified in all patients. Again the HI slope coincided with onset of ejection in all patients. We were unable, however, to establish a correlation between beat to beat variations in d^3Y/dt^3 with those in $d\dot{Q}/dt$.

Another example of Bcg and velocity is given in a patient with aortic insufficiency (AI) in figure 2. The Bcg is seen to be unusual to the extent that the HIJK complex is extremely short in duration, which may be explained by an excessively high pulse wave velocity.

The results in the five patients with the flow studies are summarized in table I and figure 3a. Plotted are the values of $d\dot{Q}/dt$ computed from the HI slope (equation 1) vs. the observed values. Each point represents the mean values in each patient, averaged over many beats. The standard deviations are indicated by bars. It is seen that except for the patient with AI, the points lie very close to the identity line; deviations from the identity vary from 2 to 16% (table I). The deviation for the patient with AI is more than 100%, but the assumed value for c of 4 m/sec is very likely to have been in error.

An example of Bcg and aortic root pressure was shown on a normal patient in the previous study [1]. Simultaneity of HI slope with onset of pressure rise was found then and confirmed in the present study.

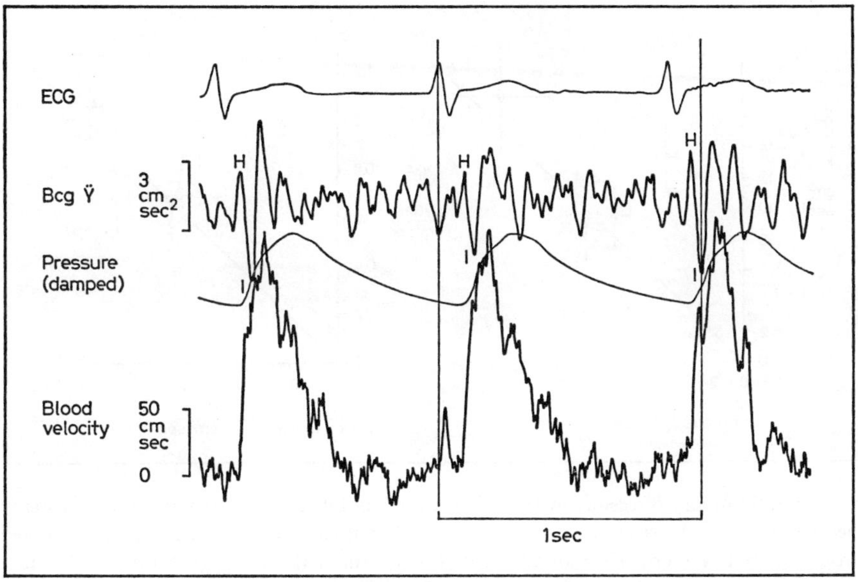

Fig. 1. ECG, Bcg, pressure (damped, not used) and blood velocity in aortic root in a 64-year-old woman (Wa.) with mitral insufficiency.

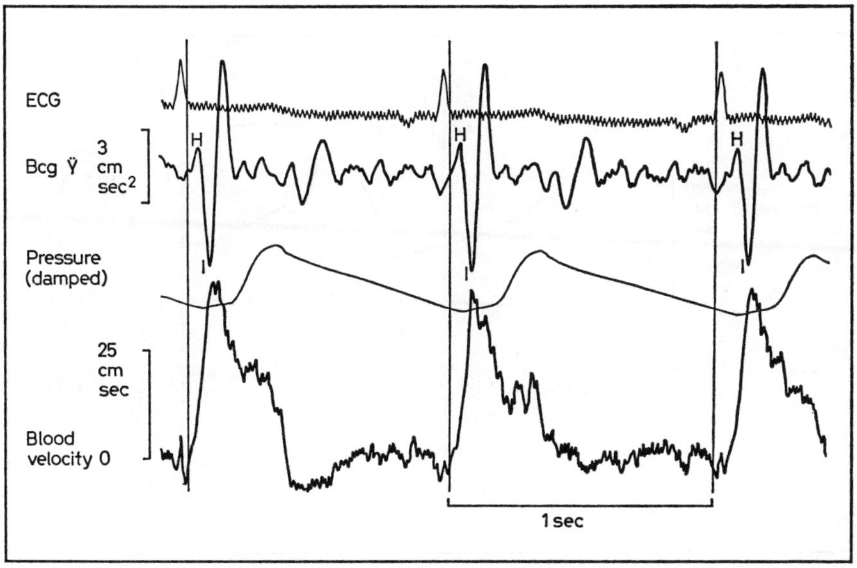

Fig. 2. ECG, Bcg, pressure (damped, not used) and blood velocity in aortic root in a 39-year-old woman (Ro.) with aortic insufficiency.

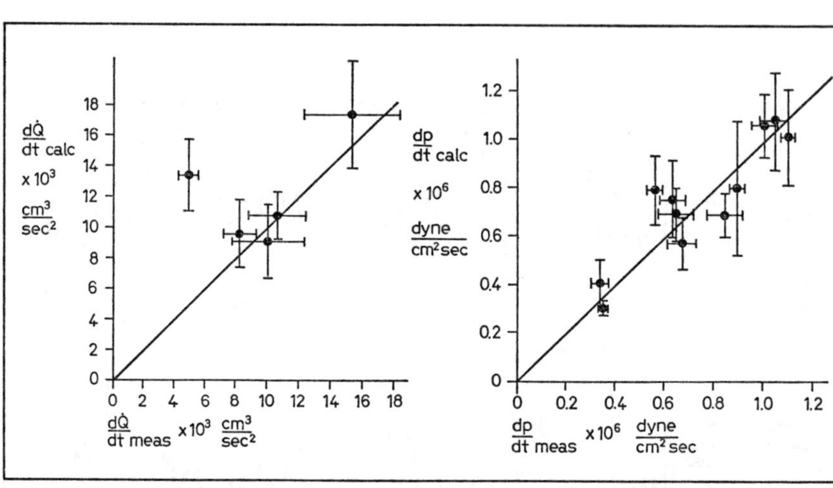

Fig. 3. Summary of results in 16 patients. Each point represents an average over many heart beats in each patient. The bars indicate 2 standard deviations. *a* dQ̇/dt calculated from equation 1 (vertical), plotted vs. dQ̇/dt measured (horizontal). *b* dp/dt calculated from equation 2 (vertical), plotted vs. dp/dt measured (horizontal). Drawn in are the identity lines.

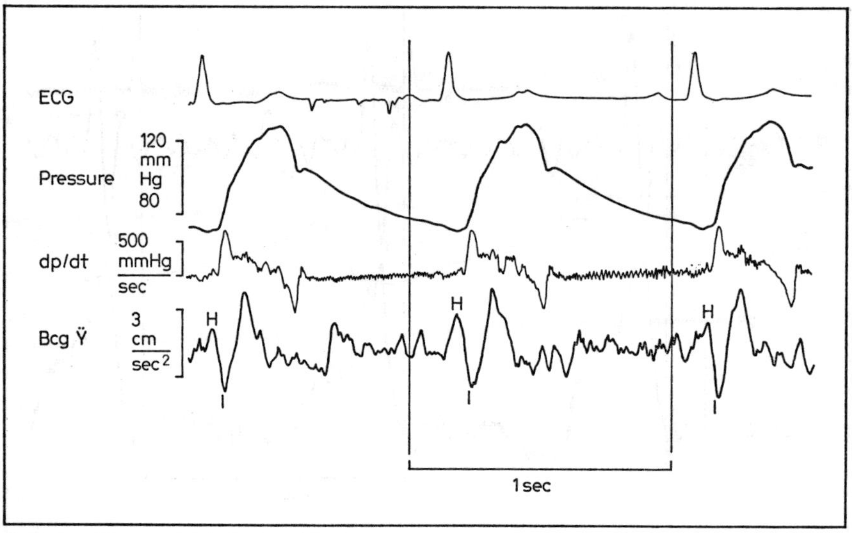

Fig. 4. ECG, aortic root pressure, dp/dt and Bcg in a 60-year-old man (Ja.) with coronary artery disease.

Table I. Summary of flow results

Patient	Age years	Sex	Height m	M kg	p_s/p_d mm Hg	HR min^{-1}	CO l/min	CI $\frac{l/min}{m^2}$	S cm^2	α degr.	$d\dot{Q}/dt$ meas.-calc. $\times 10^3$ cm^3/sec	Deviation %	Diagnosis
Wr.	45	m	1.73	75	145/85	64	5.4	2.9	5.5	20	8.2– 9.6	16	ASCAD; LV apical akinesis
Ro.	39	f	1.52	37	130/57	66	2.6	2.1	5	25	5.5–13.4	> 100	AI
Pf.	41	f	1.52	64	130/78	64	4.4	2.7	4.5	35	10.0– 9.1	9	LV apical akinesis
Wa.	64	f		42	108/65	74	8.0		5.5	40	10.6–10.8	2	RHD, MI
Bk.	24	m	1.83	85	150/100	74	10.4	5.0	6	30	15.3–17.4	13	cardiomyopathy; syst. hypertension

Table II. Summary of pressure results

Patient	Age years	Sex	Height m	M kg	p_s/p_d mm Hg	HR min^{-1}	CO l/min	CI $\frac{l/min}{m^2}$	S cm^2	α degr.	dp/dt meas.-calc. mm Hg/sec	Deviation %	Diagnosis
Re.	28	f	1.60	61	135/80	88	7.0	4.5	5	25	265–225	16	normal, abnormal ECG
Do.	39	f	1.54	45	106/70	68	6.7	4.9	5	35	820–760	8	normal
Co.	51	m	1.80	88	130/80	72	7.8	3.7	9.5	35	255–300	17	CAD
Gu.	42	f	1.67	63	100/65	108	8.8	5.2	8	25	420–590	34	normal
Jo.	55	m	1.77	92	130/80	78	6.8	3.3	6	25	470–560	22	CAD
Ba.	67	m	1.88	90	170/90	68	7.6	3.5	8	20	500–425	14	ASCAD; LV apical akinesis
Mc.	51	m	1.72	71	155/76	68	5.1	2.8	5.5	20	775–805	4	ASCAD; LV apical akinesis, MI
Va.	30	m	1.75	59	100/70	99	9.8	5.7	6.5	25	750–790	5	RHD, MS; pulm. hypertension
Ac.	37	m	1.57	61	130/70	68	7.1	4.4	7.5	40	630–520	19	normal
Ja.	60	m	1.70	70	135/70	75	8.2	5.3	7.5	40	665–600	11	CAD; LV apical akinesis
Ma.	58	m	1.57	81	195/108	120	6.9	3.7	9	20	480–515	7	systemic hypertension

CAD = Coronary artery disease; ASCAD = arteriosclerotic CAD; LV = left ventricular; MI = mitral insufficiency; RHD = rheumatic heart disease; MS = mitral stenosis; AI = aortic insufficiency.

A sample of the pressure studies in the other nine patients is given for a case of coronary artery disease in figure 4. In general, pressure contours tend to show a much more stable picture than velocities or flows. Again we could not establish a beat-to-beat correlation between dp/dt and d^3Y/dt^3.

The results obtained in the 11 patients are summarized in table II and figure 3b. Plotted are the mean values for dp/dt, computed from the HI slope, vs. the observed mean values for each patient. Again, a very good fit of the data to the identity line is demonstrated, with deviations varying from 4 to 22% in most patients, and one with a 34-percent deviation (table II). Consistent with the stable character of the pressure contour, standard deviations in observed dp/dt (horizontal bars) are substantially smaller than those observed in HI slope (vertical bars) and $d\dot{Q}/dt$ (fig. 3a).

As stated in the Methods section, measurements were obtained during apnea at the mid-expiratory level. In a number of cases, records were also secured at the end-inspiratory position. It is known that this position often improves the shape of the Bcg in cardiac patients [STARR, personal commun.]. Indeed, we observed a considerable increase in the HI slope, but this was accompanied by neither an increase in $d\dot{Q}/dt$ nor an increase in dp/dt.

Discussion

Data of the kind described here have been obtained in man previously [4] with the pressure gradient technique of obtaining velocity. Correlation between flow acceleration and Bcg (d^2Y/dt^2) was established but no mechanism for this was demonstrated.

We have shown that the experimental data in cardiac patients of Bcg, flow and pressure fit our mathematical predictions to a satisfactory degree. However, the origin of the required factor of 3/2 is not entirely clear. It might very well have other causes than the geometrical ones discussed above, all occurring during early ejection:

(1) A transitory longitudinal movement of the ascending aorta in cranial direction, a phenomenon observed even as far away as the abdominal aorta in dogs [2]. This might, however, be partly offset by a caudal motion of the heart's center of gravity.

(2) The behavior of the ballistic transfer function of the body, whose amplitude may be larger than one at the high frequencies involved [CUNNINGHAM, personal commun.]. Fortunately, the influence on the HI slope, caused by artefactual motion of separate parts of the body, was found to be very small [5].

(3) A contribution of the right heart's ejection to the HI slope, although judged unlikely by VERDOUW [15], but worth consideration in view of the results obtained from the different respiratory positions.

(4) A more sizable contribution of terms neglected in the derivation of the mathematical relationships (equations 1 and 2), because their magnitude was estimated small [1].

Unfortunately, all of these factors are very hard if not impossible to evaluate in man and require extensive animal studies. Any trials to improve on the theory of the origin of the Bcg must await these more specific measurements. In addition, the quality of the data reported here should be improved by redesigning the velocity probe, obtaining a more stable support for the ballistobed, and acquiring Bcg records during the early stage of the lengthy catheterization procedure instead of afterward. Further, a noninvasive way to estimate the pulse wave velocity has not been devised yet. Ways of estimating the angle α were outlined before [1] but not tested yet for lack of instrumentation. Errors likely to result from not knowing its precise value are small though. Noninvasive methods to obtain the value of S are probably out of the question, but the knowledge of dp/dt is not nearly as important as knowledge of $d\dot{Q}/dt$ [2a].

The failure to find a correlation between beat-to-beat variations in d^3Y/dt^3 and those in $d\dot{Q}/dt$ in the four patients studied with the CME probe may be due primarily to the relatively large amount of noise in the velocity tracings, reflected in the large standard deviations in figure 3a. Notably, in the patient studied with the SE probe the signal to noise ratio was much more favorable and we did find such a correlation.

The noise in the CME probe may be primarily caused by catheter whip and perhaps a sensitivity of the signal to probe orientation, both of which problems are less severe in the stiffer SE probe. However, because of difficulties faced with placing the latter probe in the aortic root via the brachial artery route, we decided in favor of the more manageable CME instrument.

Noise undoubtedly is also present in the Bcg tracing, obtained on the less-than-ideal support consisting of the fluoroscopy table. This can be improved only at very high cost.

We must remember though that beat-to-beat variations may also exist in the other variables entering in equations 1 and 2, especially in cross-sectional area. This may explain the absence of correlation in all of the pressure studies.

The cause for the large deviation found in the patient with AI is tentatively sought in an excessively high value for c in the ascending aorta. Aortic insufficiency usually entails an increased stiffness of the aorta and this would indeed increase the pulse wave velocity [2]. On the other hand, the measured value for $d\dot{Q}/dt$ of 5.5×10^3 cm^3/sec may represent an underestimate in view of the error inherent in the dye dilution method for low cardiac outputs (2.6 l/min).

Considerable deviations from the mathematical prediction were reported also in the previous study of dp/dt in the face of AI [1]. It must be concluded that the relationships (equation 1 and 2) should not be used in the presence of aortic valvular disease.

The observations on the effects of breath-holding position raise the possibility that it may have a strong effect on the aortic properties (c and S), alluded to previously [1]. But also the effect of altered venous return and right heart ejection may play an important role.

Bearing these comments in mind, we may conclude that the mathematical relationships derived do predict experimental data very well. Thus, in the HI slope of the Bcg we have a noninvasive way of computing the value of maximal aortic $d\dot{Q}/dt$ during onset of ejection which has been demonstrated to be a very sensitive index of myocardial contractility.

Summary

Sensitive indices of myocardial contractility derived from the blood flow during onset of ejection were expected to be quantitatively reflected in the early complex of the Bcg. Two mathematical relationships between the HI slope of the Bcg and maximal flow acceleration and pressure derivative in the ascending aorta, which had been derived previously, were tested in 17 patients during cardiac catheterization. Experimental data were found to fit the mathematical predictions very well although some limitations are indicated. It is concluded that in the Bcg we have a noninvasive tool of assessing myocardial contractility in a quantitative fashion.

Acknowledgements

The author wishes to thanks Drs. J. C. SHELBURNE and J. H. MANCHESTER for their help in the experimental part of this study, and Dr. A. P. FISHMAN for his counsel and encouragement.

References

1 BAAN, J.; MANCHESTER, J. H., and SHELBURNE, J. C.: A quantitative relationship between the HI slope of the head-foot Bcg and the initial acceleration of flow in man;

in JACKSON Circulatory assist and ballistocardiographic studies. Bibl. cardiol., vol. 29, pp. 55–69 (Karger, Basel 1972).

2 BAAN, J.: Transverse impedance in arteries: animal experiments related to wave transmission theory; Ph. D. Thesis, Univ. of Pennsylvania, Philadelphia (University Microfilms, Ann Arbor, Mich., 1970).

2a BAAN, J.; KAHL, F. R.; FLINT, J. F., and SZIDON, J. P.: Peak acceleration of aortic flow as an index of myocardial contractility (Abstract). Circulation *46*, Suppl. II: 45 (1972).

3 BRUTSAERT, D. L.; CLAES, V. A., and SONNENBLICK, E. H.: Velocity of shortening of unloaded heart muscle and the length-tension relation. Circulat. Res. *29:* 63–75 (1971).

4 FOX, S. M., III; WARBASSE, J. R.; CRAWFORD, R. B.; GREENFIELD, J. C., JR., and SCARBOROUGH, J. R.: Studies of the instantaneous ascending aortic blood velocity in intact man relative to the acceleration ballistocardiogram (Abstract). Amer. J. Cardiol. *8:* 302 (1961).

5 FRANKE, E. K.: Body dynamics and ballistocardiogram; in JACKSON Circulatory assist and ballistocardiographic studies. Bibl. cardiol., vol. 29, pp. 102–106 (Karger, Basel 1972).

6 LUISADA, A. A.: in ALTMAN and DITTMER Respiration and circulation. Biological Handbooks, pp. 416–417 (Federation of American Societies for Experimental Biology, Bethesda 1971).

7 NOBLE, M. I. M.; TRENCHARD, D., and GUZ, A.: Left ventricular ejection in conscious dogs. I. Measurement and significance of the maximum acceleration of blood from the left ventricle. Circulat. Res. *19:* 139–147 (1966).

8 NOBLE, M. I. M.: Problems concerning the application of concepts of muscle mechanics to the determination of the contractile state of the heart. Circulation *45:* 252–255 (1972).

9 NUTTER, D. O.; NOBLE, R. J., and HURST, V. W., III: Peak aortic flow and acceleration as indices of ventricular performance in the dog. J. Lab. clin. Med. *77:* 307–318 (1971).

10 PETERSON, K. L.; UTHER, J. B.; SHABETAI, R., and BRAUNWALD, E.: Instantaneous left ventricular tension-velocity relations obtained with an electromagnetic velocity catheter in the ascending aorta. Proc. nat. Meet. Amer. Fed. Clin. Res., Atlantic City 1972. Clin. Res. *20:* 391 (1972).

11 PARMLEY, W. W.; CHUCK, L., and SONNENBLICK, E. H.: Relation of V_{max} to different models of cardiac muscle. Circulat. Res. *30:* 34–43 (1972).

12 PARMLEY, W. W.; DIAMOND, G.; TOMODA, H.; FORRESTER, J. S., and SWAN, H. J. C.: Clinical evaluation of left ventricular pressures in myocardial infarction. Circulation *45:* 358–366 (1972).

13 POLLACK, G. H.; HUNTSMAN, L. L., and VERDUGO, P.: Applicability of series elasticity in cardiac muscle. Proc. 24th Ann. Conf. Med. Biol., Las Vegas, p. 96 (1971).

14 RUSHMER, R. F.: Initial ventricular impulse: a potential key to cardiac evaluation. Circulation *29:* 268–283 (1964).

15 VERDOUW, P. D.: Ballistics of ventricular performance; Ph. D. Thesis, Univ. of Pennsylvania, Philadelphia (University Microfilms, Ann Arbor, Mich. 1970).

Author's address: J. BAAN, Ph. D., Cardiovascular-Pulmonary Division, Hospital of the University of Pennsylvania, 3400 Spruce Street, *Philadelphia, PA 19104* (USA)

Proc. 16th ann. Meet. Ballistocard. Res. Soc., Atlantic City 1972;
Bibl. Cardiol. *32:* 94–100 (Karger, Basel 1973)

The Ultra-Low-Frequency Ballistocardiogram in a Young California Gray Whale

N. Ty Smith, E. A. Wahrenbrock and G. Maruschak

Department of Anesthesia, University Hospital,
University of California, San Diego, Calif.
VA Hospital, La Jolla, Calif.

The ultra-low-frequency ballistocardiogram (Bcg) has been recorded on an incredible array of animals, ranging from bird embryos to cattle. In one series, Juznic [1] observed that the difference between the Bcg's of mice and men is relatively small. We extended these observations to the whale, an animal which is a mammal but which exhibits considerable differences from most other members of its class.

Methods

The whale, a young California gray whale, was already resident at Sea World, Inc., San Diego. Thus problems involved with recording the Bcg were simple: assemble a special Bcg bed plus a set of electrical cables 50 feet long, coax the whale onto the bed, and ask her to lie quietly while the record was taken.

Gigi was captured on March 15, 1971, in Scammon's Lagoon, Mexico, at an estimated age of 6–8 weeks. She had been living at Sea World for 9½ months prior to our study; thus, she was almost 1 year old. By the time of the study she had reached a weight of over 5 tons, a length of 24′11″, and a maximum girth of 11′11″. The Bcg bed was a stretcher constructed from canvas and two 20′ heavy wall galvanized steel pipes 3″ in diameter (fig. 1). The total weight of 500 lb. may seem frightening to most ballistocardiographers, but is small compared to Gigi's mass. Actually, by the time it was constructed, the bed was too short. One cannot delay too long at a growth rate of ½ inch per day. Six ropes supported the poles, four at the ends, 13 feet in length, and 2 in the middle. A board inserted between the 2 middle ropes prevented them from injuring the animal. The 6 ropes were suspended by a single cable from a crane (fig. 2). During the recording, the cable was 25 ft from pulley to hook. The crane was part of a truck hoist, which was ideal for isolation from ground because of the pneumatic lift and the rubber tires. However, the truck was too small for the task assigned to it that day; when it tried to lift Gigi its front wheels left the ground. The driver jammed his truck as tightly as possible against the retaining wall of the tank. This seemed to prevent the truck from flipping into the tank.

Gigi was quartered in a tank 50 ft in diameter and 15 ft in depth, with a capacity of 200,000 gallons. Most of the water was drained from the tank to reduce her mobility and to enhance our own. She was reluctant to lie on the bed, and had to be coaxed. The coaxing process took 45 min. Gigi was a very gentle animal and fond of many of her human friends. However, one playful flick of her tail could have caused serious injury. Once on the bed, she remained surprisingly quiet, which was fortunate, since the same tail could easily have demolished our accelerometer. One readjustment of the relative position of whale and bed was required to level the bed.

Acceleration was transduced in the head-foot direction with an Endevco piezo-resistive accelerometer clamped to one of the steel poles. Lead II of the ECG was recorded using 4″ 18 g spinal needles. A 60-Hz passive notch filter and a 50-Hz low pass Butterworth filter were used on both the ECG and the Bcg. All electrical cables were supported by a rope stretched across the tank. We were not concerned about damping of the bed by the cables. Data were recorded on a Hewlett-Packard oscillograph and an Ampex FM tape recorder.

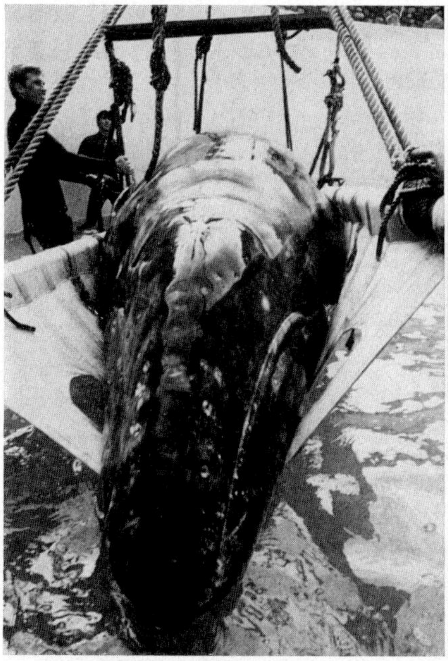

1

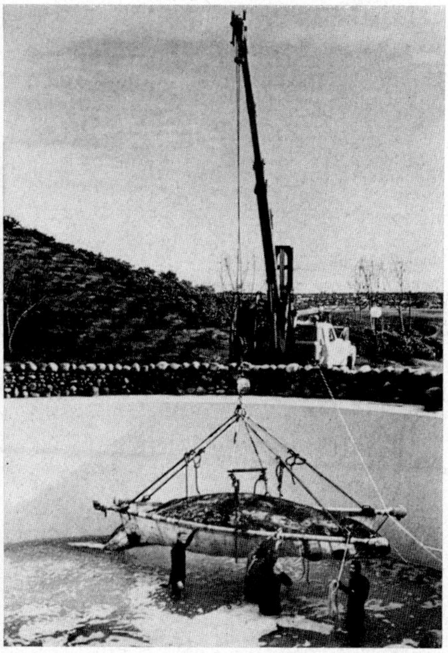

2

Fig. 1. A close-up view of Gigi in her Bcg bed. The canvas is supported by two thick steel poles. Note the board inserted between the two middle ropes to prevent their injuring the animal. Note also the left side of the mouth and the left eye of the animal.

Fig. 2. Gigi, Bcg bed, men, and hoist. The accelerometer is being attached to the right side of proximal pole, in preparation for the final lift. The truck was jammed against the retaining wall of the tank. A white rope strung across the tank supports the cables.

Results

Figures 3–5 show the Bcg recorded from Gigi. In amplitude and form, it is similar to that seen in man. Figure 6 shows the Bcg's of 3 animals – a mouse, a man, and a whale. Their similarities are more striking than their differences. For example, the IJ amplitudes in mouse and whale are 7.6 and 4.8 cm/sec².

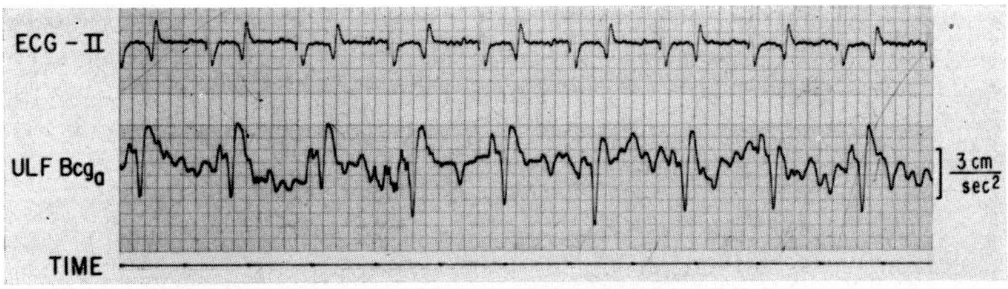

Fig. 3. ECG lead 2 and acceleration Bcg on the California gray whale. Paper speed = 25 mm/sec. The calibration of 3 cm/sec² is shown in the lower right.

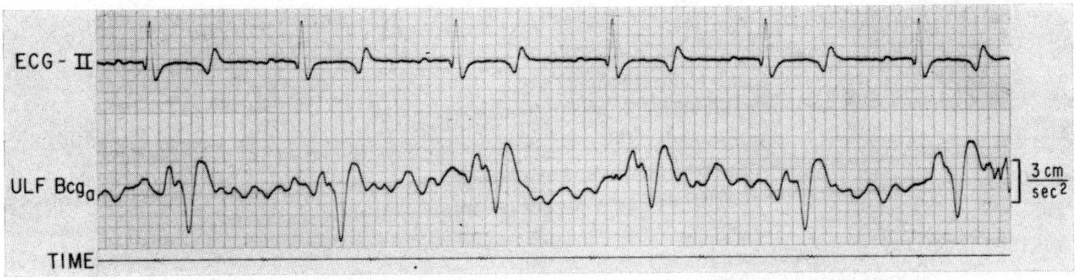

Fig. 4. The ECG and Bcg at a faster paper speed, 50 mm/sec.

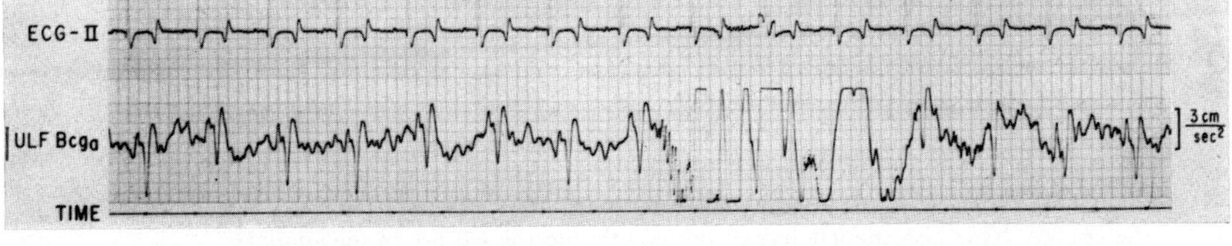

Fig. 5. The Bcg with Gigi during one breath. Paper speed = 25 mm/sec. The respiratory influence on the Bcg is considerably greater in the whale than other species. This is probably due to the necessarily rapid and large exchange.

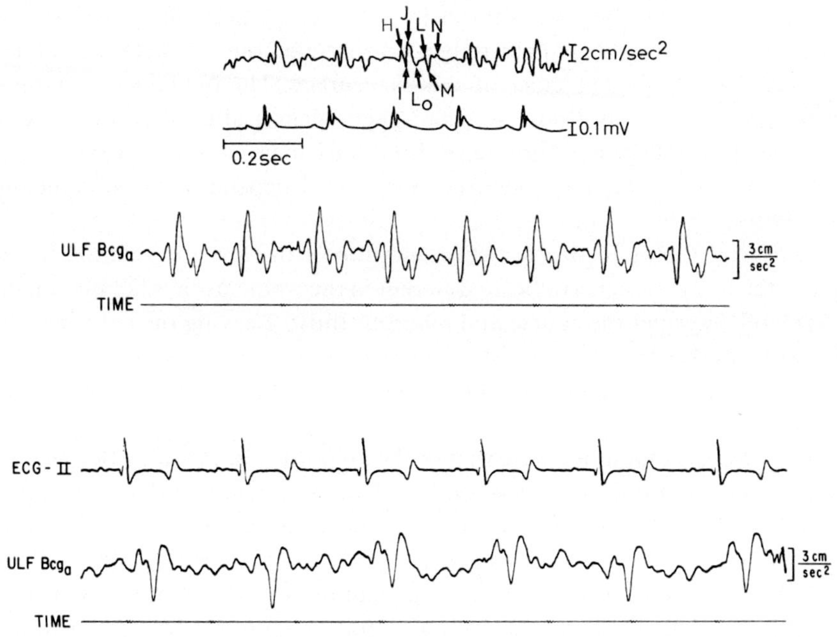

Fig. 6. The ultra-low frequency acceleration Bcg's in a 27-gram mouse (top tracing), a 73,000-gram man (middle trace) and a 4,500,000-gram whale (lower trace). The ECG's of 2 of the animals are also shown. Note the more rapid paper speed in the mouse Bcg. Considering the 167,000-fold difference in body mass, as well as the differences in body shape, amount and distribution of fat, and instrumentation, the records are remarkably similar.

Discussion

Gigi belongs to what is tragically called an endangered species. Sea World was permitted to capture her with the understanding that they would cooperate with any reasonable scientific experiment. They did cooperate, and beyond any expectation. Without their planning and enthusiastic hard work, this study would have been impossible.

The similarity in amplitude and form of Bcg's from the 3 animals is striking. This similarity holds in spite of the differences in body mass and form, amount and distribution of fat, and natural habitat.

One of the major postulated objections to the Bcg is that the amount and distribution of body fat can considerably alter the recording. This did not seem to be the case in Gigi, who had a 3.5-in. layer of blubber. It is true that the old direct-body Bcg was subject to influence by body fat. However, the ULF bed, by virtue of its light weight and strong coupling between subject and bed has eliminated most of this inaccuracy. The fundamental natural frequency of the body ('bowl of jelly' phenomenon alluded to by some in reference to the Bcg) does not depend on body mass, amount of fat, or age [2–8]. Some of the higher mode frequencies may depend on the amount and distribution of body fat.

A crucial factor in Bcg is the orientation of the aorta in relation to the rest of the body. It seems to be no different in the whale from other mammals. GREEN [9] describes the course and relations thus: 'Leaving the left ventricle, the aorta makes the characteristic left arch before passing superficially and caudally to lie just under the center of the thoracic cavity to pass through the diaphragm.'

It is obvious that if one were to plot the amplitude of the *force* Bcg against body mass, one would see a straight line. Had we integrated the acceleration Bcg to obtain velocity and displacement tracings, we would probably have seen similar constants among species.

Other constants also occur among mammals. For example, with rare exceptions, such as the giraffe, arterial blood pressure is very similar in different species [10]. One could speculate teleologically why nature has 'selected' the values for such constants. If normal pressure were higher, either the vessel walls would have to be of considerably stiffer material, or they would have to be so thick that the ratio of wall thickness to lumen would be impractical. If normal pressure were lower, perfusion through the necessarily small capillary vessels would be difficult.

Similarly, a peak-to-peak body acceleration of 2–6 cm/sec^2 (about 2–6 mg) seems to be optimum. Even at this amplitude, one can detect a slight rocking motion when lying in bed. If the acceleration is greater, as with severe aortic insufficiency, the rocking becomes quite noticeable. If the whale had a body acceleration proportionately large in relation to his mass, the motion could become uncomfortable. Why a smaller acceleration would not be feasible, or indeed why the initial ventricular impulse is necessary at all is difficult to guess.

The general outline of the form of Gigi's Bcg is very similar to that given for normal man by SCARBOROUGH *et al.* [11]. One can certainly recognize an HIJ complex and an LMN complex. We can conclude then that greater differences in amplitude and form are caused by faulty technique, such as a heavy bed and poor coupling, or by disease states, than by differences in spieces.

The major difference among the Bcg's of various mammals seems to be one of timing of the wave forms. As body size increases, the onset of the wave is delayed and the wave spreads out. Thus, in the mouse the Q-H interval ('pre-ejection period') is 27 msec and the H-J interval is 43 msec. The corresponding numbers for man are 110 and 140, for our whale 320 and 205. If we consider the tip of the H wave as the onset of ejection, we shall at worst underestimate the pre-ejection period. Certainly, the relative values can be estimated by the Q-H interval. The contribution of prolonged conduction time to these differences is probably considerable. The PR interval in Gigi was 294 msec and the QRS, 103 msec. In man the intervals are 180–200 and 80–100 msec, in the mouse they are 42 and 14 msec.

In general, heart rate and ejection time are inversely related [12]. Thus, part of the differences in intervals are due to heart rate differences. But Gigi's heart rate of 43 beats/min was not as slow as expected probably because she was excited.

A bonus of investigating an animal such as this is that ventilation frequency is so slow that it does not interfere with the recording. Gigi was relatively tachypneic at a rate of one breath every 20–28 sec. This was very fortunate since each breath demolished the recording. A whale must expire and inspire rapidly between dives. Gigi's peak instantaneous flow rate was 295 l/sec [WAHRENBROCK, E.A., unpublished data].

Gigi was released according to plan on March 13, 1972, during the northwest migration of the gray whale from Mexico to the Bering Sea. She had a radio pack on her back, so that water temperature and her position could be transmitted. When last heard from Gigi was happily heading North.

Summary

The Bcg has been recorded in an astounding array of animals, from chick embryos to cattle. It turns out that the form and amplitudes of the ULF Bcg are reasonably similar in mice and men. Therefore we took advantage of the availability of an 11-month-old 10,000 lb. California gray whale to extend the range of ballistocardiographic observations. To record a ULF Bcg, we coaxed her into a 500-lb. sling which was suspended from six 10-foot cables. The cables in turn were attached to a 24 foot cable suspended from the arm of a crane. Acceleration was transduced with an accelerometer placed on one rod of the sling. The ULF Bcg of this 5-ton animal, with a thick layer of blubber and no legs, would be considered within normal limits both in form and amplitude for man. The IJ amplitude was 4.5–5.5 cm/sec^2. This is less than twice that seen in the mouse. Thus, like arterial pressure, body acceleration is remarkably constant among mammalian species, regardless of mass.

Acknowledgements

The authors gratefully acknowledge the assistance of Sea World, Inc., San Diego, and its staff. Without their enthusiastic cooperation, this venture would have been impossible. Of particular help were Mr. BUD DONAHOO and Miss SUSAN BAILEY. The former coordinated the group effort necessary to place Gigi onto her hed. Both were close friends of Gigi, and could calm her down when no one else could. Thanks also go to Dr. DAVID KENNEY, whose ingenuity allowed the capture of Gigi.

References

1 JUZNIC, G.: The ultra-low frequency ballistocardiogram of the mouse. Bibl.cardiol., vol.26, pp.280–291 (Karger, Basel 1970).

2 BURGER, H.C.; NOORDERGRAAF, A., and VERHAGEN, A.M.W.: Physical basis of the low-frequency ballistocardiograph. Amer. Heart J. *46:* 71–83 (1953).

3 BURGER, H.C. and NOORDERGRAAF, A.: Physical basis of ballistocardiography. II. The quantities that can be measured with different types of ballistocardiographs and their mutual relations. Amer. Heart J. *51:* 127–139 (1956).

4 TALBOT, S.A. and HARRISON, W.K.: Dynamic comparison of current ballistocardiographic methods. I. Artifacts in the dynamically simple ballistocardiographic methods. Circulation *12:* 577–587 (1955).

5 TANNENBAUM, O.; VESSELL, H., and SCHACK, J.: Relationship of the natural body damping and body frequency to the ballistocardiogram. Circulation *13:* 404–409 (1956).

6 WEISSBACH, G.H.J.: Die Rolle der Tischmasse und der Wert einer zusätzlichen Dämpfung beim Elongationsballistokardiographen. Pflügers Arch.ges.Physiol. *270:* 529–535 (1960).

7 WEISSBACH, G.H.J.: Die registriertechnischen Eigenschaften des direkten Ballistokardiographen. Z.Kreislaufforsch. *49:* 626–630 (1960).

8 TISHCHENKO, M.I.: Significance of natural vibrations of the human body in shaping the ballistocardiogram (translation). Biophysics *8:* 311–319 (1963).

9 GREEN, R.F.: Observations on the anatomy of some cetaceans and pinnipeds; in RIDGWAY Mammals of the sea: biology and medicine, p.269 (Thomas, Springfield 1971).

10 Arterial blood pressure: vertebrates other than mammals; in ALTMAN and DITTMER Handbook of respiration and circulation, pp.405–413 (Federation of American Societies for Experimental Biology, 1971).

11 SCARBOROUGH, W.R.; FOLK, E.F. III; SMITH, P.A., and CONDON, J.H.: The nature of records from ultra-low frequency ballistocardiographic systems and their relation to circulatory events. Amer.J.Cardiol. *2:* 613–641 (1958).

12 WEISSLER, A.M.; PEELER, R., and ROEHLL, W.: Relationship between left ventricular ejection time, stroke volume, and heart rate in normal individuals and patients with heart disease. Amer. Heart J. *62* 367–378 (1961).

Authors' address: Prof. N.TY SMITH, Department of Anesthesia, University Hospital, University of California, 225 West Dickinson Street, *San Diego, CA 92103* (USA)

Proc. 16th ann. Meet. Ballistocard. Res. Soc., Atlantic City 1972;
Bibl. Cardiol. *32:* 101–108 (Karger, Basel 1973)

An Inherently Damped ULF Ballistocardiograph

D. M. Cunningham and T. L. Mossteller

Department of Mechanical Engineering, University of California, Berkeley, Calif.

Background

All of the current hydrostatically-lubricated air bearing ballistocardiographs utilize the same basic concept. One [1, 2], three [3], or four [4] thrust bearings support the weight of the patient by virtue of the pressure applied to the air in the space between the two bearing surfaces (fig. 1, 3). The upper bearing surface is integral with the supporting bed which then moves very freely horizontally, since the lubricating air has such a low viscosity, due to the action of the heart and blood flow dynamics. The lower bearing surface is part of the fixed supporting frame; it is sometimes flat but usually made slightly concave upwards with a radius of from 25 [2] to 90 [3] feet. In this way, the supporting bed (and the upper bearing surface[s]) not only is virtually physically isolated from ground horizontally, but has a stable equilibrium, e.g. always comes to rest at the center of the bearing when no horizontal forces are acting upon it.

Concept

The basic idea was to take advantage of the fact that a plate supported by fluid pressure would be subjected to a viscous resisting force if it was given a horizontal velocity V (fig. 1). Or, if the plate oscillated horizontally its motion would be viscously damped. Since the damping force is inversely proportional to the clearance h, which is a function of inlet pressure P_i, which in turn is a function of fluid flow rate Q, the damping force can be selected by setting the flow rate. In other words, varying the flow rate varies the clearance which varies the damping.

In the following pages the relationships between the bearing load, geometry, fluid properties, and the variables damping factor, clearance, fluid pressure, load capacity, and fluid flow rate will be developed.

Nomenclature

A	Area	T_n	Natural period of vibration
C	Damping factor	V	Velocity of bearing disk
c	$\frac{1+\varrho}{\varrho}$	v	Velocity of fluid
		W	Load on the bearing
d	Diameter	x	r/r_o = any radius/outer bearing radius
f	Frequency		
f_n	Undamped natural frequency = $1/T_n$	x_i	r_i/r_o = inlet bearing radius/outer bearing radius
h	Bearing clearance (flat-flat bearing)		
h_c	Minimum bearing clearance (flat-spherical bearing)	δ	Depth of bearing dish (difference between chord and arc of sphere)
$K_{1,2,3}$	Constants (defined in the text)	μ	Absolute fluid viscosity
k	Spring constant	ϱ	δ/h_c
L	Radius of spherical bearing	τ	Shear stress
p	Pressure	ω_n	Undamped natural frequency, radians per second
Q	Volumetric flow rate		
r	Radius		

Mathematical Relationships

Incompressible fluid flows out of a central hole (fig. 1) then radially outward under a flat circular disk. The clearance h is variable. In figure 2 are shown the horizontal forces acting on a polar element of the fluid.

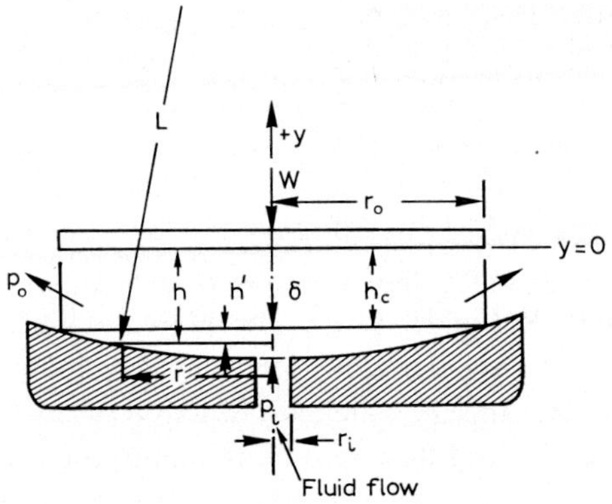

Fig. 1. Flat-spherical bearing geometry.

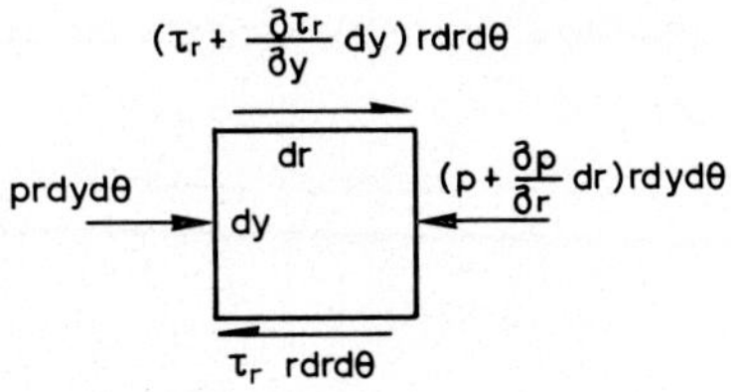

Fig. 2. Polar coordinate element of fluid.

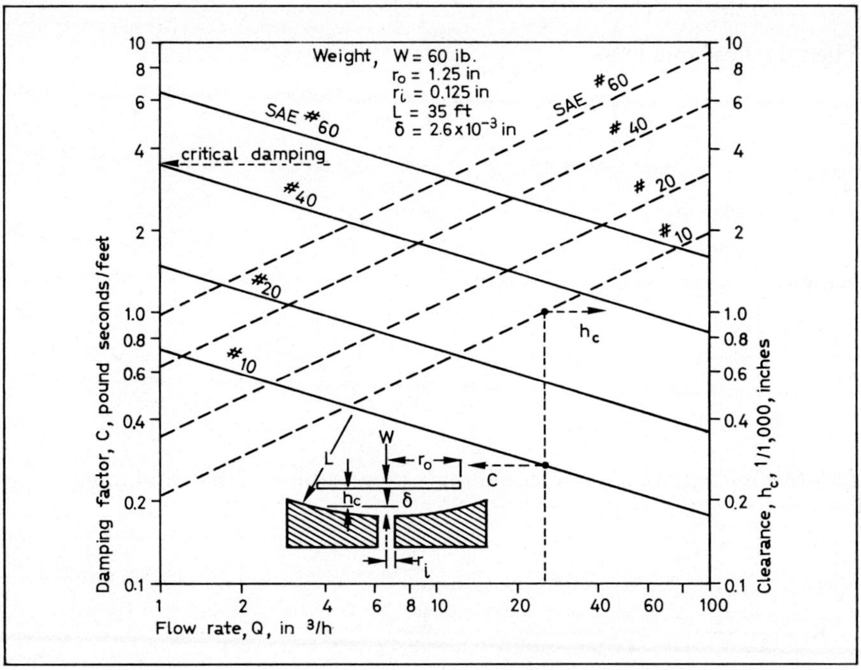

Fig. 3. Design curves for the flat-spherical bearings.

For the case of steady flow, these forces add up to zero:

$$\frac{\partial p}{\partial r}\,\mathrm{rdrdy}\theta\delta = \frac{\partial \tau_r}{\partial y}\,\mathrm{rdrdy}\theta\delta$$

or

$$\frac{\varrho q}{\partial r} = \frac{\partial \tau_r}{\partial y}\,. \tag{1}$$

Fluid shear stress and absolute viscosity are related by

$$\tau_r = \mu \frac{\partial v}{\partial y}, \frac{\partial \tau_r}{\partial y} = \mu \frac{\partial^2 v}{\partial y^2}; \tag{2}$$

so

$$\frac{\partial p}{\partial r} = \mu \frac{{}^2 v}{\partial y^2}. \tag{3}$$

Integrating twice and using the boundary conditions that velocity v = 0 at y = 0 and -h,

$$v = \frac{1}{2\mu}\frac{dp}{dr}(y^2 + hy) \cdot \tag{4}$$

Then the flow rate Q is

$$Q = \int_A vdA = 2\pi r \int_{-h}^{0} vdy = \frac{\pi r}{\mu}\frac{dp}{dr}\int_{-h}^{0}(y^2 + hy)\,dy \tag{5}$$

or

$$Q = -\frac{\pi r h^3}{6\mu}\frac{dp}{dr}, \tag{6}$$

but now,

$$h = h' + h_c \tag{7}$$

or

$$h = h_c + \delta\,[1 - (\frac{r}{r_0})^2] \cdot \tag{8}$$

Substituting equation 8 into equation 6, separating variables and integrating,

$$Q = \frac{\pi\delta^3}{6\mu}\frac{p_i - p_0}{K_2}, \tag{9}$$

where

$$K_2 = \frac{1}{4c(c-1)^2} - \frac{1}{4c(c-x_i^2)^2} + \frac{1}{2c^2(c-)} - \frac{1}{2c^2(c-x_i^2)} + \frac{1}{2c^3}\log\left(\frac{1}{x_i^2}\frac{c-x_i^2}{c-1}\right) \tag{10}$$

with

$$x = \frac{r}{r_0}, x_i = \frac{r_i}{r_0}, \rho = \frac{\delta}{h_c}, c = \frac{1+\rho}{\rho}, \tag{11}$$

$$p = p_0\left\{1 + [\frac{p_i}{p_0} - 1]\left[\frac{K_l - \frac{1}{4c(c-x^2)^2} - \frac{1}{2c^2(c-x^2)} - \frac{1}{2c^3}\log\left(\frac{x^2}{c-x^2}\right)}{K_2}\right]\right\}, \tag{12}$$

where

$$K_l = \frac{1}{4c(c-1)^2} + \frac{1}{2c^2(c-1)} + \frac{1}{2c^3}\log\left(\frac{1}{c-1}\right). \tag{13}$$

The bearing load capacity is

$$W = \pi r_i^2 p_i - \pi r_0^2 p_0 + \int_{r_i}^{r_0} \int_0^{2\pi} p\, dA, \tag{14}$$

where

$$dA = r dr d\theta \cdot$$

Substitute p = f(x,h,δ) from equation 12 into equation 14 and integrate, whence,

$$W = \pi r_0^2 (p_i - p_0) \frac{K_4}{K_2}, \tag{15}$$

where

$$K_4 = \left[\frac{2c - 1 - 2cx_i^2 + x_i^4}{4(c-1)^2 (c - x_i^2)^2} \right] \tag{16}$$

or

$$p_i - p_0 = v \frac{K_2}{K_4} \cdot \tag{17}$$

From equations 9 and 15

$$Q = \frac{W\delta^3}{\mu 6 r_0^2 K_4} \tag{18}$$

Substituting

$$\rho = \frac{\delta}{h_c} \text{ and } c = \frac{1+\rho}{\rho}$$

and letting

$$x_i^2 = \left(\frac{r_i}{r_0}\right)^2 \simeq 0,$$

the flow rate

$$Q = \frac{2Wh_c^3}{3\mu r_0^2} \left[\frac{(1+\rho)^2}{2+\rho}\right] \cdot \tag{19}$$

For a linear velocity distribution between surfaces, the basic expression for the damping factor is the same as for a uniform clearance bearing,

$$C = \frac{\mu A}{h} \tag{20}$$

Substitute the value of h from equation 20 into equation 6 and,

$$Q = -\frac{\pi r h^3}{6\mu} \frac{dp}{dr} = -\frac{\pi r \mu^3 A^3}{6\mu C^3} \frac{dp}{dr} \tag{21}$$

Separate variables, so

$$\int_{r_i}^{r_o} \frac{dr}{r} = \frac{\pi\mu^2 A^3}{6C^3 Q} \int_{p_o}^{p_i} dp\,,$$

whence

$$\log \frac{r_0}{r_i} = \frac{\pi\mu^2 A^3}{6C^3 Q} (p_i - p_0)\,, \tag{22}$$

substituting equation 15 in equation 22

$$C = \mu^{2/3} A \left[\frac{W}{6r_0^2 Q \log (\frac{r_0}{r_i})} \frac{K_2}{K_4} \right]^{1/3}, \tag{23}$$

or

$$C = \frac{\mu K_5}{h_c} \left[\frac{K_2}{K_4} \cdot \frac{2+\rho}{(1+\rho)^2} \right]^{1/3}, \tag{24}$$

where

$$K_5 = \frac{A}{[4 \log (\frac{r_0}{r_i})\,]^{1/3}}\,. \tag{25}$$

A family of curves for the flat-spherical bearing was obtained (fig. 3) for the following situation:

load per bearing, $W = 60$ lb.,
lower bearing dish radius, $L = 35$ ft,

whence

$\delta = 0.0026$ inches, for $f_n = 0.15$ Hz,
upper bearing, outside radius, $r_o = 1.25$ inches
inside (inlet) radius, $r_i = 0.125$ inches.

The single parameter varying from curve to curve is viscosity of the oil selected, given as the SAE[1] number.

Discussion

To make use of figure 3 the desired damping coefficient is selected and a suitable oil viscosity chosen. This sets the required flow rate which finally determines the nominal bearing plate clearance, h_c. For example, choose a damping factor, $C = 2.28$ (corresponding to 0.65 critical damping; a com-

[1] Society of Automotive Engineers.

promise between minimum overshoot and no harmonic distortion). Selecting an SAE 40 oil, the flow rate required is 4.0 in^3/h which produces a clearance of 0.00125 inches – a reasonable value. Using only the SAE 40 oil, by varying the flow rate via a variable – speed, constant – displacement pump from 1 to 100 in^3/h, the damping factor would range from critical damping to 0.24 critical. Meanwhile, the clearance would vary from 0.00062 to 0.00590 inches.

This range of clearances is quite realizable, with possibly two qualifications: (1) the tolerances on the shape of the bearing surfaces must be an order of magnitude less than the minimum clearance in order to allow the assumed radial fluid flow in the bearing and for the lower 'dish' to perform its pendulum-like function (say ± 0.00005 inches, a reasonable requirement); (2) if the clearance is too great the upper bearing plate in its 'horizontal' motion may not follow the lower dished contour – even to the extent of becoming unstable, e.g., moving completely off to one side. The latter case is notably apparent when air (or other gas) is used as the lubricant. However, these problems are greatly minimized when a high viscosity lubricant such as motor oil is used.

In practice, a variable volume flow rate pump would be used to supply the liquid lubricant to the bearings. The outflowing lubricant would be collected from a ring around the lower halves of the bearings and sent to a reservoir. After passing through a filter it would be supplied again to the pump.

The spacing of the three air bearings on the existing ULF Bcg was chosen to maximize the stiffness of the aluminium honeycomb bed. This is not necessarily the best spacing for rotational (about the z axis) damping of the bed when a liquid lubricant is used. It is a simple exercise, once the translational damping has been set, to choose a bearing spacing which will give the required rotational damping. Alternatively, a compromise spacing could be used.

Conclusions

(1) It is theoretically quite feasible to combine in a single set of bearings the features of horizontal bed isolation and variable viscous damping.

(2) By this scheme damping factors from ¼ critical to critical can be obtained using a single oil (SAE 40). Associated clearance would be acceptable.

(3) Rotational damping can be chosen to be the same as translational or different by the expedient of varying the bearing spacing.

Summary

By controlling the flow rate of a viscous lubricating oil, variable horizontal damping can be achieved in the three dished supporting thrust bearings. The bed still swings – as if on a long pendulum. Vertical support and horizontal motion damping are combined in one system, avoiding the additional complication of an add-on damping system as required previously when the nearly frictionless air bearings were used. The new system eliminates the need for house air, nitrogen bottle, or vacuum cleaner blower, but requires the addition of an oil pump and oil recirculating system. Only electrical power need be supplied from an external source to this otherwise completely self-contained system.

References

1 MARTIN, B.O.: Measuring the heart's kick. Time *28:* 59–60 (1961).

2 HARRISON, W.K.: Two new forms of ultra-low frequency ballistocardiograph. Proc. 11th annu. Meet. Ballistocard. Res. Soc., Atlantic City 1966. Bibl. cardiol., vol. 19, pp. 13–18 (Karger, Basel 1967).

3 CUNNINGHAM, D.M. and SMILEY, P.C.: An air bearing ballistocardiograph. J. appl. Physiol. *16:* 755–758 (1961).

4 BAAN, J.; MANCHESTER, J.H., and SHELBURNE, J.C.: A quantitative relationship between the H-I slope of the head-foot Bcg and the initial acceleration of flow in man. Proc. 15th annu. Meet. Ballistocard. Res. Soc., Atlantic City 1971. Bibl. cardiol., vol. 29, pp. 55–69 (Karger, Basel 1972).

Authors' address: D.M. CUNNINGHAM and T.L. MOSSTELLER, Department of Mechanical Engineering, University of California, *Berkeley, Calif.* (USA)

Proc. 16th ann. Meet. Ballistocard. Res. Soc., Atlantic City 1972;
Bibl. Cardiol. *32:* 109–114 (Karger, Basel 1973)

A Look at the Fourier Spectrum of the Ballistocardiogram[1]

E. K. FRANKE

Laboratory of Biophysics, Department of Physics, University of Cincinnati, Cincinnati, Ohio

Introduction

Fourier analysis of the ballistocardiogram (Bcg) is a well-established method in the investigation of various problems related to ballistocardiography, as for instance the frequency response of ballistocardiographs, the effects of the dynamics of the human body on the Bcg, or the elastic properties of blood vessels. The Fourier spectrum of the Bcg has a simple relationship to the 'Bcg impedance', which may be defined by the relation

$$F(n\omega_H) \cdot Z_B(n\omega_H) = B(n\omega_H), \tag{1}$$

where $\omega_H = 2\pi \cdot$ (cardiac cycle in seconds^{-1}), $n = 1, 2, 3, \ldots$, $B(n\omega_H)$ = complex Fourier Spectrum of the Bcg, $F(n\omega_H)$ = complex Fourier Spectrum of the flow (or pressure) pulse, and $Z_B(n\omega_H)$ = complex Bcg impedance.

Similar definitions have been used by VERDOUW [12] and TOMEK [11]. The 'characteristic function' of BURGER and VAN BRUMMELEN [4] is its counterpart in the time domain.

It would be a simple matter indeed to compute the impedance Z_B of an individual Bcg if a simultaneous record of F(t) were available; but this is rarely the case. Moreover, the advantage of the Bcg as a non-invasive method is lost when F(t) is recorded at the same time. But the concept of the Bcg impedance is still useful even when pulse wave information is lacking and equation 1 cannot be strictly solved; the puzzle of Bcg's with an excessively

[1] The Research reported in this paper has been supported by USPHS grant HE-12025.

large beat-to-beat variability is such an instance[2]. This type is quite common among class III and class IV Bcg's, which have a considerable diagnostic and prognostic potential [5]. Equation 1 shows that a variable Bcg can be generated by fluctuations of the pulse wave, fluctuations of the Bcg impedance, or both. Model studies of the Bcg have been carried out up to the present exclusively with constant parameters for the circulatory system and a strictly periodic pressure or flow input; they give few if any clues about the relative contributions of the pulse wave and the arterial system to non-periodic fluctuations of the Bcg pattern. In the absence of independent, simultaneous information on either F(t) or $Z_B(t)$, the problem cannot be solved rigorously. But it is still possible to appraise the situation at least qualitatively by changing the question: Assuming for the time being that Z_B is invariant in time, one can ask how much difference between two pulse waves (in the same subject and the same tracing) would be necessary to generate the two markedly different Bcg cycles. Will the pulse wave differences so found be reasonable and compatible with experimental evidence to justify the assumption of Z_B invariance? It will be shown below that the conclusion is unavoidable that Z_B can undergo substantial non-periodic fluctuations in addition to its well-known respiratory variability.

Method

We will now try to show how the concept of the Bcg impedance, in combination with the Fourier spectrum of the Bcg, can be employed to obtain a qualitative estimate of the pulse wave difference which would be required to explain the difference of two corresponding Bcg cycles *if Z_B were constant*[3]. From a large number of tracings[4], parts of records were selected which were suitable for our stated purpose. Two cycles of one of these Bcg records, $B_1(t)$ and $B_2(t)$, are shown in figure 1. The following series of steps is then carried out: First, a reasonable pulse wave pattern $F_1(t)$ is chosen *arbitrarily*. The adopted pattern is shown in figure 2; it is identical to the one employed

[2] A simultaneous record of Bcg and aortic pressure and flow, which has been obtained by BAAN [1], came to the author's attention after completion of this investigation. BAAN's records show the coexistence of a regular pulse wave and a very irregular Bcg very distinctly.

[3] It is self-evident that care must be taken to compare only Bcg cycles in the same respiratory phase.

[4] The records were kindly provided by DONALD C. FISCHER, M.D., Director of Medical Education, Good Samaritan Hospital, Cincinnati, Ohio.

by VERDOUW [12] in the simulation of Bcg's by an electrical analog. Next, the spectra of $F_1(t)$ and of $B_1(t)$ are computed. Finally, $Z_{B1}(n\omega_H)$ is found by equation 1. *We shall now assume that Z_{B1} is an invariant* of the circulatory system, with the reservation that the respiratory phase is properly considered. If this premise is accepted, another pulse wave corresponding to the second Bcg cycle shown in figure 1 can be computed, using the previously determined value of Z_{B1}. To do this, one has only to find $F_2(n\omega_H) = B_2(n\omega_H)/Z_{B1}(n\omega_H)$ and then to perform a Fourier synthesis to obtain the presumptive $F_2(t)$. While it is readily admitted that this function is not the actual flow pattern, it will nevertheless provide a graphical demonstration of the difference between the two pulse waves which would be necessary to generate $B_1(t)$ and $B_2(t)$ under the hypothesis of Z_B = const.

Results

The result of this computation is shown in figure 3. The pattern of $F_2(t)$ is unacceptably different from the pattern of $F_1(t)$; two pulse waves which can generate Bcg's like $B_1(t)$ and $B_2(t)$ would have to be drastically different

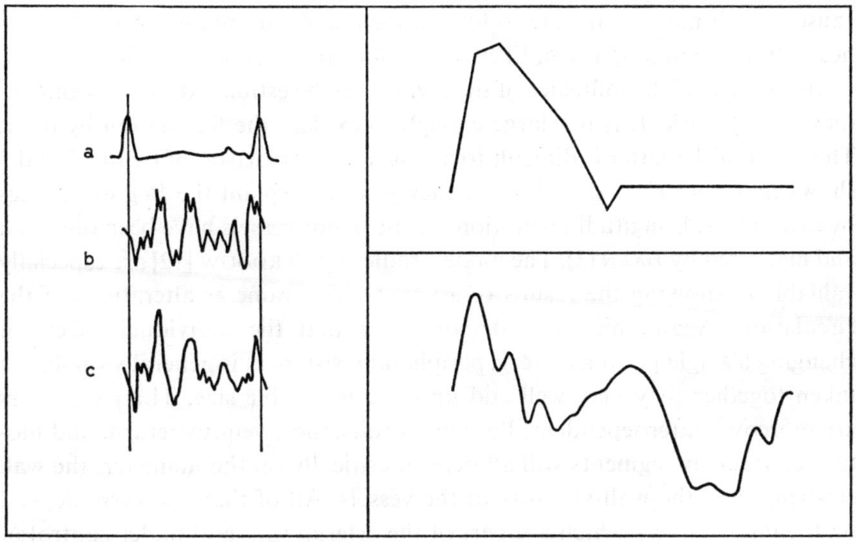

2

1 3

Fig. 1. ECG (a), Bcg 1 (b), and Bcg 2 (c).
Fig. 2. Pulse wave pattern $F_1(t)$ (1 cycle).
Fig. 3. Pulse wave pattern $F_2(t)$ (1 cycle).

indeed if an essentially invariant impedance is postulated. Other initial choices of $F_1(t)$ will lead to similarly unrealistic consequences. Identical computations were made for a considerable number of selected Bcg pairs; the resulting pulse wave patterns are always at variance with all available experimental evidence.

Discussion

The author has gone to great length in trying to find pulse wave records of the required degree of variability in the literature and among long records obtained during cardiac catheterization, but none were found. Since very irregular Bcg's are very common among patients in more advanced stages of a variety of circulatory impairments, pulse waves of similarly irregular configuration should occur frequently, but they do not.

As a consequence, the conclusions are unavoidable that Z_B itself must contribute substantially to the variability of the Bcg and that the time constant of its variation is relatively short, perhaps in the order of a few seconds. (A time constant on the order of one respiration cycle will suffice to prevent the return of the Bcg to an identical pattern after one respiration cycle.) The causes which may contribute to fluctuations of Z_B are many. Motion of the heart itself are among them, likewise small changes in flow acceleration and ejection period. The influence of the former can be estimated from NOORDERGRAAF's [8] work. It is not large enough to explain the fluctuation by itself. The effect of the latter is difficult to assess, but comparison of figures 1 and 3 shows that both should be large if they were to explain the Bcg differences by themselves. Longitudinal motions of the major vessels have been observed and measured by BAAN [3]. The model studies by VERDOUW [12] are especially valuable in showing the results of a variety of parameter alterations of the circulation. Again, his work demonstrates that the individual effects of changing a single parameter (e. g. peripheral resistance) is generally small, but taken together they may well add up to considerable size. The parameters are moreover interdependent. Peripheral resistance, venous return, and motion of vascular segments will all depend critically on the diameter, the wall elasticity, and the wall viscosity of the vessels. All of these, in turn, depend on the muscle fibers which are part of the arterial wall and under control of the parasympathetic nervous system. The elastic properties of the fibers of the arterial wall will permit active muscular control of the diameter and the elastic response in smaller vessels. McDONALD [7] has estimated an upper limit of the vascular diameter of about 1 mm for vessels which could be affected by muscular activity. Of recent attempts to determine the elastic properties of vessels *in vivo* [2, 6, 9, 10], those by PETERSON *et al.* [10] can be evaluated for contributions of muscular activity. They conclude that 'the mechanical properties ... undergo large changes involving the production of mechanical work by some structure within the vessel wall. It is probable that the structure which does work upon the vessel wall and its contents is the smooth muscle of the wall.' In their paper, as in the others, the contributions of the muscle fibers are included in the overall value of the complex elasticity. However, figure 10 of their paper shows large fluctuations of the elastic and viscous moduli when recorded after an intravenous injection of epinephrine. This can be interpreted as a regulatory phenomenon; if so, it must be mediated by the muscle fibers. The period of the fluctuation can be read from the same figure and is about 8 sec in the average, but a close inspection shows occasional rapid changes of the elastic modulus by as much as 10% within 1 sec; this is short enough to be compatible with observed Bcg variability.

Clearly, more information is needed about the vascular dynamics *in vivo.* What is known, however, is not inconsistent with a measure of active peripheral vascular control of the Bcg[5]. It still remains a mystery why the abnormal Bcg should so much more frequently be accompanied by large beat-to-beat variability than the normal one, a variability which must be attributed to variation of Z_B, according to our computations. Disorganization of vascular control in such cases should, perhaps, not be excluded as a hypothesis to explain these phenomena.

Summary

One of the more puzzling aspects of many abnormal Bcg's is their large beat-to-beat irregularity, even when cardiac cycles in the same respiratory phase are compared. This variability cannot be attributed solely to fluctuations of the pulse wave pattern. This has been demonstrated in this investigation on the basis of Fourier spectra of such Bcg's and the concept of the Bcg impedance. It serves to emphasize the fact that the Bcg is the result of an intricate interplay between the heart and a very dynamic circulatory system which incessantly adapts its parameters to changing homeostatic demands. This aspect of the circulation has not always found the attention it deserves, perhaps because analytical descriptions and computer models of the circulatory system must use fixed parameters to be feasible.

[5] There exists a body of older literature concerning the now discarded concept of a 'peripheral heart', but most of it is based on observation with instrumentation which is inadequate by modern standards.

Acknowledgements

The author is indebted to DONALD C. FISCHER, M.D., Director of Medical Education, Good Samaritan Hospital, Cincinnati, Ohio, who provided the Bcg's for this research; to Dr. JAN BAAN, Department of Medicine, Hospital of the University of Pennsylvania, who contributed helpful criticism; and to MARGRIT (Mrs. ERNST K.) FRANKE, who undertook the labor of programming and computation.

References

1 BAAN, J.: The HI-slope of the ballistocardiogram used to compute indices of myocardial contractility in man; in FRANKE Proc. 16th ann. Meet. Ballistocard. Res. Soc., Atlantic City 1972. Bibl. cardiol., vol. 32, pp. 83–93 (Karger, Basel 1972).

2 BAAN, J.; IWAZUMI, J.; SZIDON, J. P., and NOORDERGRAAF, A.: Intravascular area transducer measuring dynamic local distensibility of the aorta. J. appl. Physiol. *31:* 499–503 (1971).

3 BAAN, J.: Transverse impedance of arteries: animal experiments related to wave transmission theory; Diss. University of Pennsylvania, Philadelphia, Pa. (1970).

4 BURGER, H. C. and VAN BRUMMELEN, A. G. W.: A physicist's view on the possibilities of measurement of stroke volume by means of physical methods using ultra-low frequency Bcg; Lille med., 3e série, No. spécial, pp. 27–31 (1964).

5 FISCHER, D. C.: Use of the ballistocardiogram to assess surgical risk; in HARRISON Ballistocardiographic and clinical studies. Proc. 14th annu. Meet. Ballistocard. Res. Soc., Atlantic City 1970. Bibl. cardiol., vol. 27, pp. 21–24 (Karger, Basel 1971).

6 GOW, B. S. and TAYLOR, M. G.: Measurements of viscoelastic properties of arteries in the living dog. Circulat. Res. *23:* 111–122 (1968).

7 McDONALD, D. A.: Blood flow in arteries, p. 173 (Williams & Wilkins, Baltimore 1960).

8 NOORDERGRAAF, A.: Further studies on a theory of the ballistocardiogram. Circulation *23:* 413–425 (1961).

9 PATEL, D. J. and AUSTEN, W. G.: Impedance of certain large blood vessels in man. Ann. N.Y. Acad. Sci. *115:* 1129–1139 (1964).

10 PETERSON, J. H.; JENSEN, R. E., and PARNELL, J.: Mechanical properties of arteries *in vivo*. Circulat. Res. *8:* 622–639 (1960).

11 TOMEK, I.: A new approach to Bcg simulation; in JACKSON Circulatory assist and ballistocardiographic studies. Proc. 15th annu. Meet. Ballistocard. Res. Soc., Atlantic City 1971. Bibl. cardiol., vol. 29, pp. 92–101 (Karger, Basel 1972).

12 VERDOUW, P. D.: Ballistics of ventricular performance; Diss. University of Pennsylvania, Philadelphia, Pa. (1970).

Author's address: ERNST K. FRANKE, Dr.-Ing., Department of Physics, University of Cincinnati, *Cincinnati, OH 45221* (USA)

Proc. 16th ann. Meet. Ballistocard. Res. Soc., Atlantic City 1972;
Bibl. Cardiol. *32:* 115–119 (Karger, Basel 1973)

Relationships between the Quantitative Ballistocardiographic Characteristics and the Functional Indices at Graduated Work Load

Z. TREFNÝ, V. SELIGER and S. BARTŮŇKOVÁ

District Health Centre, Prague, and
Faculty of Physical Education and Sport, Charles University, Prague

In previous experiments we studied the response of the circulatory system to graduated physical load using quantitative ballistocardiography [1]. In this paper we will report on the relationships between the quantitative ballistocardiographic characteristics [2] and the functional indices at graduated work load.

The ballistocardiograph used had a total mass of 7.2 kg and a natural frequency of 1,000 Hz when loaded by a mass of 100 kg (very high frequency type) [3]. The apparatus was calibrated so that the amplitude of 1 cm equals the force of 1 N. The work load was performed by using the bicycle ergometer with an electric braking system (60 rpm). Three submaximal work loads (1.0, 1.5, and 2.0 W/1 kg of body weight) lasted 6 min each, and the working periods were followed by 1-min rest. The maximal work load was performed up to exhaustion of the experimental person (in average 4.4 min, 3.5 W/1 kg). At rest, prior to the first submaximal working period and at the end of each work load the heart rate, pulmonary ventilation, O_2 uptake and other indices were measured. The ballistocardiographic measurements began 5–10 sec after the end of the rest and of each working period. The amplitudes (HI, IJ, JK) were measured and expressed in units of force (N) [1]. In order to describe the changes of the heart activity, we introduced the systolic force $\overline{F}$ (mean value of the HI-, IJ- and JK-forces) and the minute cardiac force $\overline{MF}$ ($\overline{F} \cdot HR$) [2].

The experimental group (table I) was formed of 12 boys of the average age of 12.3 years. According to the indices of growth and physique our experimental group corresponds to the average Czechoslovak population [4]. From our results (table II) we can summarize the following conclusions.

In our subjects the systolic force $\overline{F}$ and the minute cardiac force $\overline{MF}$ rose regularly until the average values of 0.066 N/kg (± 0.017) and 12.12 N/kg · min (± 3.143), respectively, were reached (fig. 1). The correlation between the ballistocardiographic characteristics and the functional indices was consid-

Table I. Physical characteristics of experimental subjects

	x̄	SD
Number of subjects	12	–
Age, years	12.3	0.4
Body weight, kg	41.0	6.6
Body height, cm	151.9	7.3
BSA, m^2	1.32	0.13
BMR, kcal/1 h · 1 m^2	42.5	0.1
Body fat, %	17.0	4.5
LMB weight, kg	33.9	4.7
VC, ml	2,910	340
Hand grip, kp		
Right	20.0	4.1
Left	17.9	3.1
W 170, W	87	25
W 170/kg, W	2.1	0.6

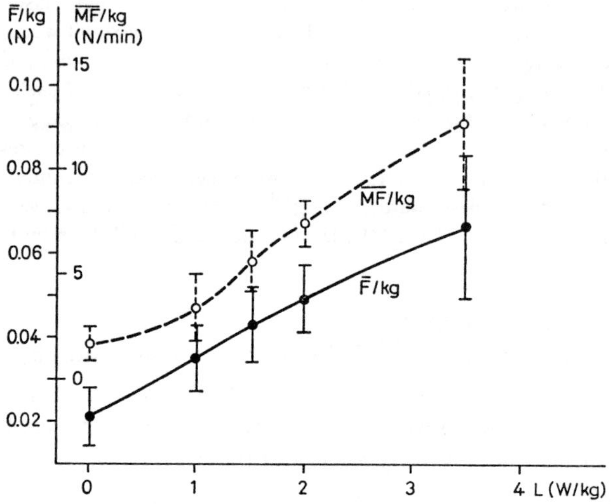

Fig. 1. Relationship between the systolic force $\overline{F}$/kg, the minute cardiac force $\overline{MF}$/kg and the graduated work load (L).

Table II. Followed quantitative ballistocardiographic characteristics and functional indices at rest and at graduated loading on the bicycle ergometer

	Rest		Submaximal load						Maximal load	
			1		2		3			
	$\bar{x}$	SD	$\bar{x}$	SD	$\bar{x}$	SD	$\bar{x}$	SD	$\bar{x}$	SD
Work load, W	0.0	0.0	41.1	6.3	62.3	9.8	82.0	12.8	142.2	18.8
Work load, W/kg	0.0	0.0	1.002	0.017	1.518	0.061	2.000	0.058	3.512	0.492
Heart rate	83.3	10.3	129.0	14.0	147.2	14.9	168.3	16.1	198.9	10.3
Pulmonary ventilation, l	10.51	2.94	27.89	4.82	33.74	5.93	40.36	6.59	73.93	13.87
Respiratory quotient	0.95	0.25	0.93	0.21	0.91	0.06	0.95	0.07	1.16	0.06
Oxygen uptake, l	0.248	0.050	0.804	0.121	0.993	0.175	1.144	0.192	1.716	0.254
Oxygen uptake, ml/kg	6.07	0.87	19.72	2.18	24.29	2.91	27.95	2.39	42.00	3.29
Pulse oxygen, ml	3.05	0.86	6.28	1.04	6.81	1.33	6.82	1.11	8.63	1.23
$\bar{F}$/kg	0.021	0.007	0.035	0.008	0.043	0.009	0.049	0.008	0.066	0.017
$\overline{MF}$/kg	1.715	0.843	3.424	1.614	5.567	1.488	7.402	1.125	12.112	3.143

ered to be significant if it was on the 1- or 5-percent level. The ballistocardiographic characteristics at rest and at the first submaximal load were not in correlation with the ballistocardiographic characteristics at the maximal load. The ballistocardiographic characteristics at the second and third submaximal load were correlated positively with those at the maximal load but not with those at rest. A negative correlation of the balistocardiographic characteristics was found with the height, the body weight, and the weight of the lean body mass, but not with the fat percentage calculated from ten skin fold thicknesses measured with a caliper. At some loads the ballistocardiographic characteristics were correlated negatively with the maximal pulmonary ventilation reached. The oxygen uptake per kg body weight was not in correlation with the ballistocardiographic characteristics.

Our experiments show that at higher body weight and at higher weight of lean body mass the values of systolic force $\overline{F}$ and minute cardiac force $\overline{MF}$ are relatively smaller. This fact is probably connected with higher biological age and with better adaptation to physical work in subjects with higher weight of lean body mass. The absence of correlation of the ballistocardiographic characteristics with the oxygen uptake at the maximal load is connected with high participation of the anaerobic metabolism at maximal load.

Summary

Using a bicycle ergometer we followed with 12 boys of the average age of 12.3 years the relationships between the quantitative ballistocardiographic characteristics ($\overline{F}$, $\overline{MF}$) and the functional indices during the graduated work load. $\overline{F}$ and $\overline{MF}$ are relatively smaller at the higher body weight. There is no correlation between $\overline{F}$ and $\overline{MF}$ with O_2 uptake in the maximal load due to the high participation of the anaerobic metabolism.

References

1 TREFNÝ, Z.; WAGNER, J.; SELIGER, V., and BUCHBERGER, J.: Force measurements in adults and schoolchildren by quantitative ballistocardiographical method; in DEUCHAR Ballistocardiography. Proc. 6th Europ. Congr. on Ballistocardiography, London 1957. Bibl.cardiol., vol.21, pp.152–156 (Karger, Basel 1968).

2 TREFNÝ, Z. and SELIGER, V.: The use of quantitative ballistocardiography for the measurement of the circulatory system in the graduated work load; in SCARBOROUGH Ballistocardiography and circulatory function. Proc. 12th annu.Meet.Ballistocardiograph.Res.Soc., Atlantic City, N.J. 1967. Bibl.cardiol., vol.20, pp.106–109 (Karger, Basel 1968).

3 Trefný, Z. and Wagner, J.: A quantitative ballistocardiograph; in Noordergraaf and Pollack Ballistocardiography and Cardiac performance. Proc. 11th annu. Meet. Ballistocardiograph. Res. Soc., Atlantic City, N.J. 1966. Bibl. cardiol., vol. 19, pp. 19–25 (Karger, Basel 1967).

4 Seliger, V. *et al.*: Physical fitness of the Czechoslovak 12- and 15-year-old population. Acta paediat. scand, suppl. *217:* 37–41 (1971).

Author's address: Dr. Z. Trefný, District Health Centre, Faculty of Physical Education and Sport Charles University, Prague (Czechoslovakia)

Subject Index